P9-AGP-441

# DATE DUE

| | | | |
|---|---|---|---|
| 00 29 '95 | | | |
| | | | |
| | | | |
| | | | |
| | | | |
| | | | |
| | | | |
| | | | |
| | | | |
| | | | |
| | | | |
| | | | |
| | | | |
| | | | |
| | | | |
| | | | |
| | | | |

# HEALTHY COMPUTING

This book introduces you to the various ways in which frequent use of a computer for long periods may be detrimental to your health—and what you can do to protect yourself. It is not a substitute for obtaining professional advice for potential or existing health problems. Every individual is different, and so are the circumstances in which we do our computing. Consequently, the authors and publisher cannot be responsible for how you apply or interpret the information in this book. Use it as a guide to healthier and happier computing, but seek professional advice for your specific needs, and especially before undertaking any major diet or exercise program.

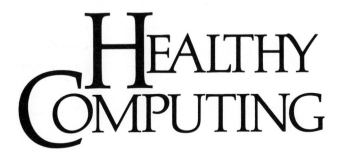

# HEALTHY COMPUTING

## RISKS AND REMEDIES EVERY COMPUTER USER NEEDS TO KNOW

Dr. Ronald Harwin &
Colin Haynes

**amacom**

**American Management Association**

ies.
Department,
lanagement Association,
135 West 50th Street, New York, NY 10020.

This publication is designed to provide accurate and authoritative information in regard to the subject matter covered. It is sold with the understanding that the publisher is not engaged in rendering legal, accounting, or other professional service. If legal advice or other expert assistance is required, the services of a competent professional person should be sought.

*Library of Congress Cataloging-in-Publication Data*

Harwin, Ronald.
    Healthy computing : risks and remedies every computer user
    needs to know / Ronald Harwin, Colin Haynes.
        p.    cm.
    Includes index.
    ISBN 0-8144-7766-6 (pbk.)
    1. Video display terminals—Health aspects.   2. Computers—
Health aspects.     I. Haynes, Colin.    II. Title.
RC965.V53H37    1991
616.9'8—dc20                                           91-53058
                                                           CIP

Printing number

10 9 8 7 6 5 4 3

# Contents

# Foreword

Health problems related to operating computers demonstrate how rapidly technology develops and how slowly humans adapt to changes required by these innovations. Fortunately, there are simple, natural, and practical solutions to many of the physical and mental stress problems that arise from the way that we force ourselves to live and work. This book is rich in such solutions. They should be taken seriously, even if many appear to be simple "low-tech" answers to complex "high-tech" issues.

My life as a researcher is devoted to two very complex areas of science. I study how the brain and central nervous system function, particularly in relation to addictive substances. Recently I have also devoted much time to the problems of nutritional deficiencies among African people. In both these spheres, tangible benefits to alleviate human suffering have come from applying natural measures with a minimum of complexity.

For example, we have helped thousands of recovering alcoholics through their withdrawal symptoms by replacing expensive, complex—and potentially dangerous—drugs with therapies using nitrous oxide, a natural substance that has existed since the beginning of life on earth. Also, we have identified how a variation in traditional cooking habits and the addition of small quantities of one of the most common substances—lime—to flour can alleviate suffering among millions of Africans with dietary deficiencies.

In this, his latest book to help general readers understand complex technical and scientific issues, Colin Haynes has again cut through the technical jargon, the misinformation, and the contradictory arguments of vested interests. He and Dr. Ronald Harwin have penetrated the problems created by human interfacing with computers and assembled practical solutions. Sometimes the advice on changing how we work at the keyboard may sound almost too simple and easy to be effective, but it is no less valid for that. The American Management Association is to be congratulated on tackling such an important subject in such a practical way, bringing to all of us who use computers (or who supervise computer operators) information that we can put to good use.

Dr. Mark Gillman
Consultant, Albert Einstein Medical School,
    New York City
Director, South African Brain Research
    Institute

# *Preface*

Ken Goehner is a professional writer of computer articles, and a victim of the very technology from which he makes his living. One day he woke up to a nightmare—his hands were paralyzed.

As an expert in computers and, like most journalists, a professional skeptic, Ken is well-qualified to give an impartial report on how the techniques advocated in this book helped him to solve his problem.

> I often work long and continuous hours, only to collapse from exhaustion. Some time ago, I was working to meet a deadline—it was my second all-night computing session of the week. After I finished my story, I sent it off by electronic mail and went to bed. When I woke up, I found that both my hands were partially paralyzed.

> The next couple of months were a nightmare. I was in severe pain, incapable of work, and racking up thousands of dollars in medical bills. And the most I got out of this encounter with modern medicine was a month on painkillers— an experience similar to being buried headfirst in cement!

> I then met Dr. Ronald Harwin, who explained to me that my wrist pain and paralysis did not come from a single traumatic accident, but from years of repeated "postural and functional microtrauma." Put simply, microtrauma is repeated low-level

aggravation of a body part caused by using it improperly in ways for which it was not designed. These tiny microinjuries add up over the years to a full-blown injury that may have serious consequences.

Much to my relief, Dr. Harwin's treatment provided almost immediate results. Within three days, my hands started to feel stronger and my pain had decreased. In a matter of weeks, I had regained virtually full use and total feeling in my right hand. Three months later, I was virtually back to normal, with 95 percent use of my left hand also.

No amount of work or money is worth the agony I endured. Fortunately, others can avoid a fate similar to mine if they understand how long-term computer use can damage health. We all need to be aware of the simple preventive steps that can be taken to avoid microtrauma and other computer-related injuries.

Georgia Rowe is another victim of the computer, diagnosed as suffering from bilateral carpal tunnel syndrome.

After using computers for twelve years, I had begun to experience some frightening symptoms: intense pain in my hands, wrists, and forearms, with a numb and tingling feeling in my hands.

At first these symptoms appeared only while I was working at the computer and would subside at the end of the day. After a few weeks, however, they persisted for hours after I stopped working. Eventually, the symptoms didn't go away at all, even if I didn't work for days.

The doctors I consulted easily diagnosed my condition. After all, injuries like mine have become increasingly common in computer users. But they were at a loss to tell me exactly how it had happened, or what I could have done to prevent it.

One doctor said I was probably just genetically predisposed to this type of injury. Another said it was a result of overuse of my hands—in other words, I had been working too hard.

But I knew other people who worked hard at their computers and did not suffer in this way.

The more I tried to find out about my condition, the less I learned. The only things the doctors agreed on was my need for surgery. Without it, they said, I risked permanent nerve damage and loss of feeling in my hands. Although not completely convinced, I agreed reluctantly to undergo surgery.

Four months later, I was still in so much pain that I couldn't return to work. My doctor assured me that the pain would begin to recede, but could not predict when I might expect this relief.

Then a friend gave me an article on computer health by Dr. Harwin. I contacted him and began treatment at his clinic.

Within two weeks, the degree of pain in my hands and arms had been reduced to a manageable level. After about a month, I began to be free of pain for long periods following treatment.

In addition to treating my symptoms, Dr. Harwin worked with me to identify my work habits, posture, and other factors that might be responsible for aggravating my condition. He taught me specific techniques that I could use at work and at home to alleviate my painful symptoms.

Those self-help techniques are deceptively simple and may be incorporated easily into any work routine. They encourage us to be responsible in managing our most precious possessions—our bodies and our health.

Ken Goehner's and Georgia Rowe's stories are not uncommon. It is not unusual for anyone to feel stiff and tired, or perhaps suffer a headache or eye discomfort, after working at a computer for several hours. But it is not *normal*—and it is certainly *unhealthy*—to feel this way. Ignore these symptoms at your peril, for there is a good chance that you will end up with an injury that will damage both your professional and personal life—an injury as serious as those which afflicted Goehner and Rowe.

If you work on computers, you can avoid such dismal prospects by learning simple techniques to help you feel good while you work, maintain a high productivity level, and prevent the type of injury that has caused such pain and threatened the careers of Ken Goehner, Georgia Rowe, and hundreds of thousands of other innocent victims.

This book will help you identify the causes of computer-related health problems and take practical steps to prevent or overcome them. We call the simple tips that you will find throughout the book Quick Fixes. They may not always be enough, so we also discuss more complex techniques and remedies that have worked for many computer users. We urge you to read all we have to say in the following pages, not just skim to your symptoms or think that one or two of our Quick Fix suggestions provide the complete answer. Using a computer can affect your health in varied and complex ways, and these effects often result from a combination of factors rather than from one simple cause-and-effect incidence.

In Chapter 1, we present an overview of how computing can be hazardous to your health. Then we move on to look at both your body and your computer system in more detail so that you can work with your system in a healthier way. Specific chapters are devoted to the major problems associated with computers, such as eye ailments, headaches, repetitive stress injuries, and emotional stress. We also discuss the importance of exercise, diet, and the proper desk and chair as solutions to major computer health problems. The final chapter of the book is devoted to a discussion of the controversial topic of radiation so that you can analyze your degree of potential risk and take the measures you feel are necessary to protect yourself.

If you are an employer or manager, you can use this book as a cost-effective training tool by making it readily available to your data processing staff. Having your staff read it might also reduce your exposure to liability actions. Even the most conscientious employer cannot achieve a healthy computing situation alone because so much of the responsibility rests with the actual operator. Legal considerations aside, every employer has a moral obligation to encourage employees to act to prevent computing-related health disorders, and not wait until problems become apparent. That also makes good business sense, since people are the most valuable resource of most organizations. Prevention is better than cure in all health matters, especially in computer-related problems, because there is so much that can be done inexpensively to prevent problems from occurring.

# Introduction

# Computing Can Be Hazardous to Your Health (An Overview)

Working at a computer keyboard can be very hazardous to your health. The major occupational injuries and diseases of the 1990s will be suffered by those who spend much of their working lives—and perhaps their leisure hours as well—at a keyboard.

Computer-related health problems include:

- Repetitive stress injury (including carpal tunnel syndrome and tendonitis)
- Headache
- Tinnitus (noise in the ears, such as ringing, buzzing, and roaring)
- Head, neck, and lower back problems
- Stress-related disorders
- Eye dysfunction and sight deterioration
- Emotional/mental health problems
- Pregnancy complications

The bad news for over 60 million computer users and their employers around the world is that computing poses health problems that can be physically and economically crippling. Users are getting sick, and employers are being exposed to enormously expensive medical costs, liability claims, and disruptions to their operations. Typical costs to a company for each afflicted employee are around $10,000 in medical expenses and lost productivity. In some cases, they can top $100,000 if legal liability for industrial injury becomes an issue. Computer-related health problems collectively cost American business several billion dollars each year.

When the San Francisco Board of Supervisors in late 1990 introduced pioneering legislation to protect computer operators, the city's business community estimated that compliance by 1992 could cost them $100 million initially. Many companies calculated that it would be cheaper for them to leave their hearts in San Francisco and move their businesses elsewhere. But, of course, now every local authority is having to face up to the need to protect employees within its jurisdiction. Just as regulations to control smoking and race and sex discrimination in the workplace have been introduced nationwide, so inevitably will be legislation to protect computer operators.

So expect furniture that will adjust easily, video monitors with low electromagnetic emission levels, regular work breaks at least every two hours, and special training and health monitoring programs all to become mandatory.

But that need not be bad news. If both business and employees adopt reasonable, sensible attitudes toward protecting the health of computer operators, the savings achieved from reduced medical costs and increased productivity should more than compensate for any expenditure on new hardware and changed working habits. The really good news in this book is that the cause of virtually all pain at the keyboard can be either eliminated or drastically reduced by comparatively simple, low-cost measures.

## Unrecognized Dangers

You may not be suffering yet, but you can become sick and injured disturbingly quickly, before you realize what is happening. Even just a few hours a day working at a computer may lead to some of the health problems we listed earlier. The causes may be obscure and difficult to diagnose. A symptom, such as soreness or a sharp pain in one part of the body, may be caused by computer work that involves a completely different part of the body.

The impact need not be physical, but may also be mental or

emotional in character. For example, the noise your computer makes may be hurting you. Sound at or beyond the extremes of human hearing can make you ill. Researchers in Indiana have found evidence that the high-pitched tone emitted by some video display monitors can generate headaches and other stress-related problems.

At the other end of the sound spectrum there is a type of noise called infrasound, which is below the frequency levels that are audible to humans. Scientists know comparatively little about infrasound, but it has been linked with motion sickness. The dizziness and nausea that you may feel in a boat, plane, or car may stem from the very low frequency sound generated by the engine and the structure of the vehicle vibrating. Infrasound vibrations may be how some animals and humans can sense that an earthquake is about to occur.

Extreme levels of infrasound can cause internal bleeding. The levels that we are exposed to when working with computers and other types of office machinery are much less than that, but they may still make us feel ill. One of the authors first experienced this with an old IBM golf ball typewriter mounted on a metal desk. He could not understand why he became tense and slightly nauseated as soon as he sat down at that desk. Then, by a process of elimination, he discovered

R/

## Quick Fix #1

Noise can be very stressful when you are computing—even noise that you don't consciously hear, like high and low frequency sounds that are beyond the audible range. Check to see if your equipment could be a source of stressful noise.

Laser printer and computer cooling fans are major suspects. Try moving the units or insulating them from a surface such as a desk top that may be amplifying the sound. Also check out possible sources of stressful sound in your working environment. Some music when played continuously in the background can be very stressful and directly affect your mood. That applies to high opera as well as to heavy metal!

that the symptoms appeared only when the electric typewriter motor was switched on. The problem was solved by putting the typewriter on a thick foam pad, which eliminated the vibrations.

When he moved from typewriters to computers several years later, he experienced similar symptoms with an IBM-PC clone in a metal case and with a particularly noisy fan. Things got a lot better when he mounted it on thick foam rubber pads, and the problem disappeared altogether when he invested $20 in a stand so that the computer could be removed from the desk and be stood vertically on the floor, almost out of both sight and hearing.

So if you are experiencing symptoms of stress and nausea when computing, try Quick Fix #1.

## Understanding the Risk

Computer users—both those of us who earn our living with the aid of computers and the more than 30 million for whom they are a major leisure activity—are only now becoming aware that we face serious risks. That awareness is growing rapidly, particularly because this is the first occupational hazard that the media people are exposed to themselves as front-line victims, and consequently they are reporting about it. Some of the earliest and most severe cases of carpal tunnel injury have arisen among reporters, editors, and writers using electronic editing systems in newspapers and broadcasting organizations. Newspaper reporters across North America are suffering from RSI—repetitive stress injury. At the Los Angeles Times alone, over 200 of the 1,000 members of the editorial staff have sought medical help.

The problem isn't limited to journalists. Airline clerks, programmers, officer workers of all kinds, and many other categories of workers who use computers are also suffering. Together they are the first victims of what threatens to develop into an epidemic of computer-related medical problems.

Some ten states now regulate computer work, and most others are considering legislation. Many corporations are realizing the consequences of employees' not using computers in healthy ways. The Hertz Corporation had 20 percent of its data processors in Oklahoma submit tendonitis claims because of the repetitive keyboarding of car rental contracts. Nearly half of the directory assistance operators at a former

Bell company, U.S. West Communications in Denver, have filed RSI claims.

The National Institute for Occupational Safety and Health reports a rapidly increasing incidence of computing-related RSI problems, and now more than half of all U.S. workers are exposed to this type of injury. This includes most of the nation's 40 million office workers who use a computer keyboard every day. The cost to corporations can be enormous when you add together legal and medical expenses, lost time, reduced productivity, higher operator error, and other cost consequences.

Repetitive stress injuries, along with fears about radiation hazards from monitors, keep capturing the headlines. But neither is the most common adverse consequence of computer work. Badly designed computer workstations cause most medical conditions, especially those with the greatest potential to develop into chronic pain situations. Someone sitting with incorrect posture in an unsatisfactory chair with the keyboard and monitor in ergonomically unsound positions can literally become crippled.

The crippling process develops insidiously for years until, without warning, serious physical damage has resulted. Muscles go into spasms; nerves become compressed; tendons in the wrist and arm become inflamed because of excessive friction from hitting the keys up to 20,000 times an hour.

Intense concentration without regular changes of position creates a host of head, neck, and back problems—all with painful consequences. The position, adjustment, and type of monitor can cause head pain and eye disorders. Concern is mounting of the potential dangers—particularly to pregnant women—of something so simple as the incorrect positioning of video display terminals.

## Dangers to Children

We should be particularly concerned about the long-term consequences of computing on the health of our children. At a rapidly escalating rate, young people are spending long periods using computers at home and at school. There are now special programs written to amuse preschoolers and help them learn. The best of these can contribute much to a child's intellectual development, but we must be very careful of the potential for harm to young bodies still developing. The eyes and the body's skeletal structure are very vulnerable during the early years. Bad habits, particularly harmful sitting postures and unhealthy diets, can become programmed into young bodies and minds and lead to problems later on. The addictive intensity of some computer games can make young people completely unaware of physical discomfort and the trauma occurring to their bodies over long periods of time.

## Reprogramming Your Body

When you become aware of how both the whole body and its individual parts are at risk from unhealthy computing, you will recognize the prime dangers and know how to protect yourself from them. Then you can reprogram your body. Just as you can get a fresh start when your computer seizes up, so too you can "reboot" your body. To pursue the computing analogy, you can actually upgrade your physical and mental performance when working at your computer, just as you can upgrade the hardware and software to make it work faster and smarter.

You will learn that, because of the interconnecting relationships between body components, a pain in one place may be the symptom of a problem in another part of the body a considerable distance away. Your hands may hurt because of a problem in your neck, just as your printer may not function because there is a faulty connection way at the other end of the cable where it links with the serial port.

## Simple Solutions

You will be delighted to learn how often the apparently most difficult problems can be overcome by the simplest solutions.

Just breathing properly is an example of this. Millions of computer users become so engrossed in what they are doing that their breathing becomes only a shallow reflex action that brings in just enough oxygen to keep their bodies functioning. You must breathe properly at the keyboard. Open and relax your chest, bring air into your lungs and your body, and your brain will get significant oxygen boosts that increase the quality of your computing considerably. Otherwise you may be like a car running with a dirty air filter, able to achieve only a fraction of your performance capability.

---

℞

# Quick Fix #2

Yawn regularly when you are computing. Then you deliberately deploy this body reflex action to give your system a boost when it is running short of oxygen. Yawning also relaxes the eyes and the body in general. Alternatively, pause at least every half hour to breathe deeply—and *exhale fully*. Do this gently several times and you will feel refreshed.

---

## Pain-Preventing Exercises

A few simple exercises can reduce stress and combat the onset of the main hazards linked to computer operation. In spite of the nonsense often propounded about exercising, we don't believe that "there is no gain without pain." The exercises we give you in Chapter 5 are gentle and pleasant and reduce stress while they *prevent* the conditions that cause pain and dysfunction.

---

℞

# Quick Fix #3

Periodically pause, allow your hands and arms to drop down to your sides, and gently shake your hands and fingers as if you were flicking water off them. This helps to relieve tension and stress in the arms and hands, facilitate blood flow, and generally tone up these overworked computer operator's limbs and extremities.

## Right and Wrong Hardware and Software

Selecting hardware and software that is kind to your mind and your body can make an enormous difference in your overall well-being. So in Chapter 8 we brief you on keyboards and other input devices, monitors, accessories, and other computing hardware. Software that eases mental stress and strain—with consequent physical as well as psychological benefits—is covered also. Quick Fix #4 is an easy way to make many software programs far easier and less stressful.

---

# Quick Fix #4

Take a little time out to learn how to create the macros and hot key combinations that are features of many word processing and other keyboard-intensive applications programs. You can slash literally thousands of keystrokes out of a day's work by creating and using macros for frequently used instructions or text entries.

---

## Are You Sitting Dangerously?

One of the most effective ways of countering many computer-related health problems is to have ergonomically correct workstations. In Chapter 9 we compare different types of desks and chairs to find the right combination for you.

We also have some tips on how existing workstation furniture can be modified. If you are stuck with the furniture you already have, you should be pleasantly surprised at what can be done to make even the cheapest or oldest desk or chair more comfortable and healthier to work with.

Do not rush out and buy special furniture until you read Chapter 9. And don't automatically believe the advice you may have heard that expensive backless kneeling chairs are quick fixes that always work. After long, intense sitting, they may aggravate, rather than cure, *your* difficulties. However, refer to Quick Fix #5 for an ergonomic tip that can often be a big help.

---

℞

# Quick Fix #5

If the front edge of the seat of your chair presses behind your knees, you are probably restricting blood circulation to your lower legs and feet. Cramps and other problems are an almost inevitable consequence. Try a telephone directory or other foot support of similar thickness that is just enough to ease the pressure off the backs of your thighs. (If you need a foot support so that your feet touch the ground, you need to adjust or change your chair and/or your desk!)

---

You may get some good ideas from our description of the ergonomically ideal desk (see Chapter 9). One of its main features is a movable section which allows the position of the monitor and keyboard to be varied easily and quickly. This enables the operator to achieve the most ergonomically correct seated position and to change frequently to a standing position while working.

The ability to change position can reduce—sometimes even eliminate—many computer-related health problems, as well as dramatically increase productivity. A University of California research project indicated that mental productivity performance improves by as much as 30 percent when you stand.

Some work efficiency experts have given much attention to bringing everything within easy reach of a seated computer operator. That may appear to increase productivity by saving seconds here and there, but the overall health benefits of a worker's periodically changing position and alternating between seated and standing positions can be far more significant, both to the employer and the computer operator. The mobile and adjustable desk concept is ideal also for the handicapped confined to wheelchairs or beds.

In fact, there's good news throughout this book for everybody who uses computers. So let's get started by checking over the connections in your mind–body–computer relationships and reprogramming your mental, physical, and electronic systems to ensure pleasure, not pain, at the keyboard.

# Quick Fix #6

Try to organize your computer workstation—and your work activity—so that you regularly vary your position and stand as well as sit. Try moving the keyboard and monitor to a high surface and see if you are one of the many people who actually get less tired and feel more comfortable standing to work. If you have a portable computer, you can experiment with a variety of working positions. You may also raise the level of peripheral equipment that you use frequently—a printer, for example—so that you are forced to get out of your chair and stand while you attend to it.

# 1

# An Essential Principle: Work With Nature, Not Against It

By using a computer, you defy one of nature's most amazing achievements—the sophisticated coordination of natural movement. Computing—marvelous technology that is is—can affect us adversely because it is alien, even hostile, in many respects to both the physical and psychological ways we are designed to function. When computers enter our lives, we often overlook the need to retain our sense of humanity, individualism, and self-worth. Many human beings end up functioning in some respects more like a computer than human animals. The authors think it is basically wrong that we are required to adapt ourselves—physically, emotionally, or mentally—to accommodate any kind of machine, especially the increasingly important computer. It must bend to our will and needs.

There is a joke among dog fanciers that some dog owners come over time to look like their pets. Their dogs are so important to them that they begin to assume mannerisms and acquire physical characteristics that match their dog's.

It is no joke that computer users eventually display visible changes resulting from their close relationship with their machine. They may not get to look like a Mac, acquire square eyes, or assume the coloring of IBM beige, but they do tend to have distinct physical characteristics.

Try to pick out the people around you whose body shape and

language reflect the fact that they work intensely at a computer. Among the recognition features are a tendency to lean forward in their chairs, with their heads and necks extended out, unbalanced over their work. Their chests are somewhat collapsed, with their shoulders rolled in. Their eyes may be sharply focused most of the time, looking at fixed points immediately in front of them, rather than relaxed and wandering over their surroundings.

Such undesirable postures have been acquired from the rigidity and imbalance of protracted periods at the keyboard. Muscles and joints have become frozen and there is an ongoing battle with gravity, rather than a harmonious conformity with gravitational forces.

# Quick Fix #7

Take a moment to check on your working posture. Place a large mirror by your side as you work at the keyboard, or get a friend or colleague to describe how you look—even take a photograph that you can study. If you are adopting a posture that is stressed, unnatural, or uncomfortable, then immediately move or adjust your keyboard, screen, mouse, or chair to improve it.

## Lessons From the Ancient Martial Arts

The martial arts provide some superb solutions to computing-related physical problems. These disciplines have, over the centuries, refined techniques for relaxation, balance, and cooperating with gravity that can be applied to computer work.

Aikido from Japan and T'ai Chi Ch'uan from China are two traditional forms of martial arts that can teach us much about our postures and attitudes when interfacing with computers. Many of their principles of movement and body balance under the stress of confrontation can be applied directly to reduce stress and eliminate the injuries we sustain as we work at our keyboards.

The martial arts teach us that the body is designed and works best when integrated with the mind functioning within natural connectivity and interaction of its parts. We have the mobility and flexibility to perform natural tasks by means of joints and muscles that do not adapt readily to the artificially isolated movement of many computing tasks, such as repeated short, sharp keyboarding or mouse action finger movements.

You may be hurting yourself at the keyboard simply by the way you position your head or your hands. Intensive mouse use in computer-aided design or desktop publishing work over time can lead to very painful injuries. The body performs poorly and breaks down when one of its components is used repeatedly in isolation from the rest of the body, becoming overstressed, sustaining damage, and subsequently failing.

For example, the body and head and arms are balanced and integrated when we are engaged in such natural activities as walking. But when we sit at a desk for prolonged periods of time, our heads and hands tend to function in isolation from the rest of the body and so eventually become severely stressed and weakened.

As a response to the unbalanced leaning forward of the head, or the continually outstretched hands, our muscles, ligaments, and joints become injured. The brain may even fail to receive a full supply of well-oxygenated blood. One direct consequence of even a mild decrease in blood supply to the brain is tiredness, perhaps depression, leading to deteriorating performance in terms of both productivity and accuracy. That loss in quantity and quality of the computing work we are able to do may stem directly from a poor sitting position.

## Beating Our Brains

Bad computing habits can abuse our brains in many respects. We damage our brains when computing by exposing ourselves not only to unnatural hostile forces such as electromagnetic radiation and other pollutants but also to extremely high levels of emotional stress that are detrimental to the brain's electrical and chemical balance. We starve our brains of oxygen and essential fluids needed for efficient functioning, then blast them with potentially dangerous medication to ease the headaches and tension we created. The pills mask the pain so that we can continue to compute and abuse ourselves even more!

Our bodies are still genetically designed for hunting and gathering. We are not biologically designed to operate computers intensively. This evolutionary upgrade will take a very long time. So it is both unnatural and unhealthy to spend sustained periods looking at a screen and punching a keyboard.

But if we take the appropriate precautions, make adjustments in our work habits, and adopt simple, commonsense ergonomic principles at our workstations, we will then interface in a much healthier way with these very useful machines. Computers and humans can get along very well when the correct interface is established.

## Solve Many Health Problems by Moving Your Head

You can avoid many health risks by holding your head correctly when you are working. How you position your head for hour after hour at the keyboard may be the most important single factor in preventing many of the pains and other problems generated by bad computing habits.

Holding your head incorrectly will not, if you are lucky, generate any symptoms for a long time, but the damage is still being done insidiously. This slow, almost invisible development of damage to the body is like the slow, relentless damage from smoking tobacco. This is what is so dangerous about computer-related injuries. If the damage occurred quickly, we would have no difficulty recognizing the severity of the problem. When something we do today may not hit us in the form of pain or disablement for several years, we postpone doing something about it. But if you do not position your head correctly today, you could be in pain before too many tomorrows have passed.

Millions of years of evolution have given us brains that typically weigh 2.5 percent of our total body weight. Our brains are ten times bigger than those of elephants, but the anatomy of elephants, horses, and other four-legged animals makes them far better suited than human beings to have their heads hanging forward in front of their bodies in a fixed position for hours at a time. For example, a horse's shoulder bones are large and solidly attached to the rib cage and upper back of the skeleton. This allows great strength and stability for holding the neck and head out from the body.

This is accomplished by having a large surface area for the neck and back muscles to attach to and lever from, and by limiting severely the movement capacity of the shoulders so that they can act as a solid base from which the large muscles of the neck can anchor and pull.

The major muscles responsible for holding up the horse's head and neck are large and strong. When muscles of this size are anchored to the solid shoulder structure of the horse, the animal can easily hold its head out in front of its body with no injury developing.

With the human neck, this type of leverage and functional strength is not possible, because the shoulder girdle is designed to be extremely mobile in its connection to the rest of the skeleton. This allows for a great range of motion in the shoulders and neck and enables us to quickly and easily move our heads in response to visual and auditory cues. But we have lost the stability in the neck that animals still have.

It is very damaging to our muscles, tendons, and joints to hold our head hanging out over the keyboard day after day. It takes an enormously powerful muscle structure from the shoulders through the neck, with an appropriate leverage design, to hold a comparatively small head in a forwardly levering position for any significant time.

The human neck is deliberately not designed for this role at all. Yet most of us sit for hours—years—with our heads stuck forward in a very horse-like posture as we stare at the monitor display. To reduce the danger, refer to Quick Fix #8.

---

℞

# Quick Fix #8

Imagine you are a puppet, suspended on a string from the top of your head. There is a gentle pull upward on the string, making you raise your head vertically on your neck as you tuck in your chin. Square your shoulders and slightly arch your lower back. This is a natural, balanced position for prolonged computer work. Get someone to move your keyboard and monitor to help you maintain this position.

---

## Pause Regularly for a Body Audit

A little earlier you used a mirror or a colleague to get a new perspective on how you work. Now take slightly longer to conduct a more comprehensive body audit, examining your reflection in detail to see how you are using your body when working at the computer.

You may well find yourself slouched forward in your chair, with your chest collapsed, shoulders rolled in, your neck and head projected forward, and your feet in any number of stressful, cramping positions. Much of this misuse of your body is happening without your realizing it, because computing work is far more focused than normal clerical or other traditional office tasks. You focus almost exclusively on one thing—the computer screen.

A regular body audit will refocus your attention on how you use your body when you are working. Like your computer, your body is designed to function in specific ways. It is true that the human body (just like a computer) has a lot of tolerance for abuse, but if you use it incorrectly for too long, or push its limits too far, it is going to break down. And because it is much harder to repair your body than a computer, the consequences may be much more severe.

The head is implicated in so many computing-related health problems that we must keep returning to it. Slouching forward, so characteristic of the computer user, is a major cause of many computer-related health problems. Remember, the head weighs twelve to eighteen pounds, and when it leans forward for hours at a time, the muscles between your shoulders lock in contraction to hold your head up. This causes compression and decreases the blood flow in this area, resulting in injury to the tissues. They become swollen inside and exert pressure on the nerves controlling arm and hand coordination. This, in turn, weakens the functional strength and coordination of the hand. One consequence is increased vulnerability to carpal tunnel syndrome, tendonitis, and other repetitive stress injuries.

Slouching in your chair with your neck craned forward may not be causing you any serious problems—yet. Today you may end computing sessions with only a slight headache, or maybe just a stiff neck. You may not even feel anything untoward at all and so still not be aware that your head position while you work has already actually deformed your body and partially disabled you.

## Is *Your* Neck Deformed Already?

We know of computer users who have discovered only by accident that they have become deformed and disabled. One pulled a muscle in his leg when lifting his canoe out of the water after a weekend cruise. While he was receiving treatment for this obvious injury, his chiropractor gave him a general examination and found that the canoeing computerist had only 40 percent of his normal neck movement. He simply could not turn his head from side to side as normal people can. The patient had become so accustomed to the way his body had adapted to the stresses that computing placed on it that he did not realize that his head and neck movement had become very limited.

This restricted movement was sufficient for the eight hours a day he spent at the keyboard, so he did not notice it. When not working, he subconsciously adjusted to this disability by turning his upper body so that he could see behind him when walking or driving. He instinctively compensated for the lost joint mobility from long-term computing.

Such restricted head and neck movement is very common in people who have been working with computers for several years. The condition can be very difficult to treat in its advanced stages. It may require protracted soft tissue manipulation, appropriate exercise, traction, and, most important, teaching the patient proper work habits.

To see if you have this problem, look at Quick Fix #9.

---

℞

# Quick Fix #9

Stand upright with your back against a wall. Keep your shoulders touching the wall and your chin tucked in. Now try to touch the upper back of your head against the wall without moving your shoulders or raising your chin. Similarly, turn your head and gently try to touch each ear alternatively against the wall, maintaining the position of your chin and shoulders. If these movements are painful—or impossible—you must pay more attention to your computing posture, change your working position frequently, and exercise your head and neck as described in Chapter 5.

## Medication Is Not a Solution

Medication cannot offer permanent solutions to such muscle, bone, and joint deterioration; it can only mask the pain, not cure the problem. Occasionally anti-inflammatory drugs can be helpful in the short term, but unless the causes of the injury—one's work habits—are changed, the symptoms are likely to recur.

Indeed, medication can prove counterproductive by relieving the pain symptoms that should warn you to change how you work. Taking painkillers frequently may guarantee further injury. By masking the body's natural warning mechanism—pain—you silence the body's communications system advising you that it is being forced to function in an unnatural way for which it was not designed.

This situation is aggravated when unhealthy computing habits spill over into other activities. The slouched-forward posture becomes part of us and we can be frozen in this position when driving the car, watching television, sitting at a concert, or reading.

Only when our canoeist had his disability pointed out to him did he understand why, in the previous year or so, his family had become less confident when being driven by him. He subconsciously compensated at the steering wheel for his restricted head movement by not looking as frequently to one side or the other. So he was paying much less attention to what was going on in areas of peripheral vision, resulting in a couple of near-misses when he had been unaware of overtaking vehicles or pedestrians stepping off the curb.

Such habitual patterns of behavior modified to accommodate impaired body function can affect many aspects of our lives. If you find it more difficult than it used to be to turn your head and look behind you before changing lanes, and rely far more on your mirrors, you may well be adjusting to restricted head and neck movement. Another frequent symptom is discomfort and difficulty in turning to look behind you when driving in reverse.

Our computing canoeist even had trouble at the movies. He went to see a wide-screen action movie—the 1989 re-release of *Lawrence of Arabia*—and the only seats available were in the front row. When he had seen the movie years previously during its first run, he could have sat right up front and comfortably followed the action at each edge of the screen by turning his head. Now, twenty years of computing later, if he hadn't swung his shoulders as well as his head, the Bedouins on their camels would have ridden right out of his field of vision well before reaching the edge of the screen!

## A Health Warning Is Overdue

Society's experience with tobacco's dangers eliminates any excuse for the authorities' not issuing strong warnings about the potential hazards of computer use. The microtrauma damage that leads to serious illness and disability in computer users can also take five to fifteen years to develop, so specific cases are only now emerging and building into epidemic proportions. But we have no need to be ignorant that this is happening, or of the enormous potential cost to ourselves and to the business community.

According to Insurance Council estimates, when you add up medical costs, drugs, the purchase of products claiming to ease the suffering, and disability settlements, bad backs alone are costing the country over $80 billion a year. Backache is only one of many health problems that stem from computer use, so the scale of the issue is very worrying.

## Link the Causes and Effects

This book is written in a particular way to be of the greatest help to you, with quick references to problems and their solutions. However, there are several basic common causes of a variety of problems related to our interfacing with computers. It is often not easy to realize the links between them—and how they may relate directly to your particular situation. So we frequently repeat important advice, such as the need to breathe correctly or the importance of natural joint angles, in the hope that this may trigger you to recognize a particular detrimental computing habit that you may have, or offer an explanation for a problem you are experiencing that may be remedied comparatively easily.

An essential part of successful treatment for your problems is understanding why you are injuring yourself. Once you understand the cause of your problems, you can easily change your work habits and protect your health. It is a fascinating learning experience that generates immediate personal benefits.

# 2

# Eyes: Our Number One Concern

Computer users worry more about the effects of their work on their eyes than on any other aspect of their health. Such concern is only partly justified, but our eyes are so precious that it is well worth following the simple procedures that will help to protect them from the adverse effects of prolonged periods of looking at the video display on a cathode ray tube (CRT) or the liquid crystal display (LCD) most often used with portable computers.

Surveys repeatedly show that the majority of office workers rank eyestrain as their most serious concern among the hazards they are exposed to in their workplaces. The same surveys show that managers and executives tend to be less conscious about eyestrain as an issue, despite the effects on staff morale and the potential exposure to employee liability suits if action is not taken to minimize the risks. One probable reason for this discrepancy in perception between management and computer operators is that most offices are designed for traditional pen and paper work. Managers who do not use computers for long periods just do not appreciate the effects this can have on the eyes.

While medical specialists and researchers continue to argue over the impact of both the visible and invisible radiation from VDTs, there is no doubt that many eye and other health problems stem directly from the more obvious effects of using a CRT monitor for long periods.

Fortunately, you can do a great deal about these problems even if you have already begun to display symptoms of harm. In many cases, computer users have been able to rejuvenate their eyes by exercise, simple treatments, and changes in their work habits.

## Exposed and Vulnerable

Eyes are the only body organs directly exposed to the environment, so they are extremely vulnerable to any environmental hazard. Until computers appeared on millions of desk tops, our eyes deteriorated or failed mainly as a consequence of natural aging processes or physical injury. We rarely abused them at work (and it is a myth that you can permanently damage your eyes just by using them a lot in normal reading situations). But now, in the 1990s, our exposed eyes take a beating from the enormous increase in airborne pollutants, and we put them continually through a high-stress, dangerous survival course whenever we turn on the VDT and look at it for long periods.

Even if you do not live in Los Angeles, New York, London, Paris, Rome, or any other urban area with high atmospheric pollutant levels, you may still be exposed to pollution because your VDT can cause a localized increase in pollutants in the air. The effect is rather like the winds created by some tall buildings. They generate airflow in their immediate vicinity that can be very uncomfortable. In parts of Manhattan, for example, the area at the base of a skyscraper may have dust, dead leaves, and litter scurrying about the walkways and getting up your nose and into your eyes while most of the city is enjoying a comparatively still, windless day.

Your VDT creates similar effects on a much smaller scale, but because they are created within a few inches of your head—with your vulnerable eyes particularly exposed—they merit serious attention. Your VDT gets warm when it is switched on (that's why there are ventilation slots and baffles at its sides and top). The warmer air rising sucks in cooler air from below and the sides, much of it rushing past your head and eyes if you're sitting close.

This airflow can increase your exposure to passive smoking, pulling in smoke-contaminated air from neighboring workstations. If you are a smoker yourself, the air flowing toward and around your monitor can pick up minute particles of ash and other tobacco waste products from your ashtray. These may get into your eyes and cause physical abrasion and soreness. They are also the source, or at least contributors to, many other eye problems.

## A Magnet for Dust

Additional irritants accumulate around your VDT because the cathode ray tube that creates the picture produces electromagnetic fields. The VDT is, in effect, a magnet for dust-borne particles, which is why the screen gets dirty so quickly. The situation is aggravated if the main computer is acting as a support for the monitor or standing next to it—the normal configurations in most workstations. The computer's cooling fan and the electromagnetic forces generated by the CRT can attract so much dust that the computer may overheat and begin to malfunction mysteriously. For your hardware's health, it is good preventive medicine to open up the case of a PC (but not a Macintosh) and blow or vacuum away the dust every six months or so—more often in dusty environments.

As dust and other particles flow toward the screen, some of them inevitably get into your eyes, while the slow, probably imperceptible buildup of pollutants on the surface of the screen makes it more difficult to read and so contributes to more eye-stressing conditions.

## Dry Eyes

The typical office has low levels of humidity because of air conditioning, and that enhances the electromagnetic effects as well as makes it more difficult for the eye's natural lubrication system to cope. The tendency when concentrating on images displayed on a VDT is to blink far less often than is normal, so the tears, which lubricate, protect, and disinfect the eye, are unable to play their full, natural role as environmental barriers. The risk of physical damage to the eye is increased, just as would be the risk of your car's engine seizing up if you ran it without adequate oil circulating or without the air cleaner in place to filter out abrasive particles.

Many people—even those with expertise in the field—tend to play down the significance of airborne particles causing eye problems for computer users. They may feel that our exposure is no greater than that of other office workers. Little valid research has been done into this problem, and, anyway, it is not easy to differentiate between the eye problems caused by airborne pollutants and those resulting from other VDT hazards. However, we think a particularly convincing argument lies in the number of people who quickly contract facial dermatitis—rashes and other eruptive skin conditions on their faces—after working at a VDT for just a few hours. Such conditions are often accompanied by soreness of the lips and red, uncomfortable eyes.

It has been demonstrated that this facial dermatitis is attributable directly to airborne pollutants attracted to and concentrated around the VDT. The face and eyes are particularly exposed to some of these pollutant particles because the electromagnetic forces and airflow patterns generated by the CRT can actually propel them toward you. The particles drawn into the general vicinity of the VDT may be propelled out toward your exposed face and eyes.

## Efficient Eye Lubrication

You risk making matters worse if you wear mascara and other eye makeup. They can be eye irritants in their own right, especially if minute particles of powder flake off into an eye unable to flush them away because its teardrop lubrication system is not working properly. If you wear contact lenses, these physical problems may be compounded.

Dry eyes bombarded by alien particles that they are unable to flush away are very susceptible to infection, such as recurrent incidences of conjunctivitis, a particularly uncomfortable eye malady in which the eye becomes red and sore.

The eye exercises at the end of this chapter will help, but even more important is simple preventive maintenance. Just use Quick Fix #10.

If your eyes are taking a beating from physical irritants in your working environment, make a point of washing them out whenever you visit the restroom. You can use special eyewashes in squeeze bottles or in small eye baths. But be careful not to use them excessively, as some contain chemicals that may, with extensive use, inhibit the eye's natural self-cleansing and lubrication processes. It is an effect similar to the continual use of laxatives so that the bowels lose their natural, automatic functions. A safe and low-cost alternative to commercial eye cleansers is distilled water, which provides a neutral wash that can be used frequently without ill effects.

The easiest way to apply any eyewash is with a specially designed eyecup, but if one is not available then a small drinking glass will do almost as well.

---

℞

# Quick Fix #10

To stimulate tear formation and lubrication, blink regularly. Also, use tear substitutes if your eyes are dry. There are many different brands of artificial tears, and they differ considerably in their consistency. Some are very fluid and will run down your cheeks before they have had a proper chance to lubricate the eye, so you may get better results if you use artificial tears with a thicker consistency that will stay in the eye more easily. Experiment until you find a brand that suits you best and use it two or three times a day, more if the air in your working environment is particularly dry or there is a high proportion of particle pollutants in it, as will occur in a dusty place, during winds in arid, desert areas, in city centers with high traffic congestion, and near some "dirty" manufacturing operations. Be sure to choose a brand without vasoconstriction properties, as these have particular medical purposes and should not be used for general moistening of the eyes.

---

## Allergies and Infections

Be particularly careful not to introduce infection when drying or rubbing your eyes. If you do not practice basic eye hygiene, you might unjustly blame many eye problems on your VDT. Soaps and towels, even facial tissues, may contain substances that can infect or cause an allergic reaction in the eyes. You may increase your exposure if you wash your eyes more frequently without being careful about cleanliness. Cosmetics, pollen, and aerosol sprays may also affect your eyes and cause allergy symptoms, including the burning sensation so many of us experience after long hours at the keyboard. You may need to do some detective work and elimination tests to identify eye problems not necessarily attributable to the VDT.

## Environmental Causes of Eyestrain

There are many conditions in which the VDT *is* the obvious culprit. If computing is giving you serious eyestrain problems, you have lots of options, including inexpensive and easy fixes.

First, is your monitor screen positioned and adjusted correctly? In almost any office, you will find computer operators squinting at screens and stressing their eyes quite unnecessarily. In many cases this is because the workstation is laid out so that the monitor reflects excessive light from windows, lightly colored objects such as filing cabinets, walls, or partitions, or artificial light fixtures.

Most offices are actually too well lit for computer use, a problem that may be exacerbated by highly reflective white walls, curtains, and furnishings. The next time you wear a white shirt or dress, notice whether your image is reflected in the monitor screen.

We have moved into the electronic data processing age with lighting standards still applicable to working with paper. So offices tend to have illumination levels at desk surfaces that may be three or four times as bright as those preferable for viewing a monitor screen. There are two main negative consequences—glare from excessive light reflected from the screen, making the display difficult to read, and too sharp a contrast between the level of screen illumination and the ambient light or particular spots in the rest of the work environment.

You may, for example, be forcing your eyes to adjust continually between the very bright reflections of the papers on your desk and the much darker VDT screen. This can be a particular problem if you have one of those desk lamps designed for spot illumination. You concentrate a strong beam of light on your papers and flick your eyes backward and forward between them and the screen.

Even if your work does not involve continually alternating your gaze between screen and papers, brighter objects at the periphery of your vision can be stressful to your eyes. You think you are looking only at the screen, but your eyes are also having to cope with bright white light from papers positioned near the edge of your field of view, perhaps even strong light coming from the bulb of a desk lamp.

The colors of the walls and furniture may be significant factors. White walls may reflect too much light in an uncontrolled way, but a decor that is too dark may have adverse effects on mood as well as visibility. Some of the best lighting can be achieved with soft light colors, such as cream or beige.

Fixed office light, usually overhead fluorescent light and sunlight coming through the window, is the main cause of glare on the VDT. In offices where work is predominantly performed on computers, the lighting should be reappraised to move it from the paper to the electronic age. One major beneficial change is reducing the general overhead illumination and increasing specific localized lighting that can be varied easily by the individual operators at each workstation.

You may dismiss the unwanted reflections in your screen as just an annoyance. In fact, they may be causing you far more physical and emotional stress and discomfort than you realize. Even if the glare still leaves the screen image discernible, both the contrast of the display—the differentiation between light and dark areas—and its resolution, or clarity, can be seriously reduced. You are forcing your eyes to work excessively hard to cope with a display that is far below the quality that your equipment would be delivering if it didn't have to compete with the ambient light more appropriate to the traditional office.

## The Glare Problem

The main solutions are obvious. Reduce—or reposition where possible—the overhead lighting and cut down the sunlight glare by means of blinds or by moving your workstation. Cardboard hoods

---

℞

# Quick Fix #11

To zero in on sources of glare and unwanted reflections, use a mirror. Placed in front of the monitor screen, it will identify clearly the sources of reflections. By moving the mirror around, you can find the best position for your desk and monitor for reducing glare and reflections.

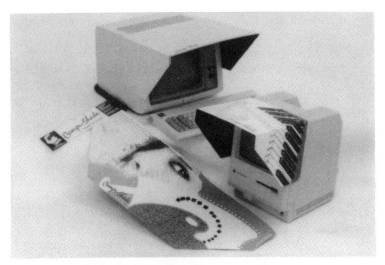

**Figure   1.** CompuShade screens.

positioned over the top and to the sides of the screen can make a big difference.

The CompuShade screens shown in Figure 1 are slick commercial versions of the makeshift cardboard hoods. Although hoods can make a dramatic improvement in screen legibility, it is best to achieve permanent lighting arrangements appropriate to computer use.

You may benefit from wearing your own version of a hood—a visor that will protect your eyes from direct exposure to glare. (Of course, this will not reduce unwanted reflections or other deficiencies in the light falling on the screen.) Do not wear polarizing or other special antiglare glasses before you have explored all the other options of eliminating the glare at its source. Remember one of the fundamental principles of healthy computing: that you adapt your computer system and its environment to *your* needs, not force yourself to make compromises to meet the demands of your equipment. Human needs come first; we should still control the machines!

## Antiglare Filters

There are now many special screens that fit over the front of your VDT display to reduce glare and ultraviolet light. They work like the quality sunglasses that help protect your eyes on sunny days by the sea, in the snow, or at high altitudes. We all know that such ultraviolet light can make our eyes sore, and some computer operators have reported symptoms similar to those they experience at the beach or out in the snow on a sunny day. Some scientific research has also suggested that there may be a link between exposure to ultraviolet light and the development of cataracts.

In addition to reducing ultraviolet light, a good-quality screen or filter can work wonders to reduce eye fatigue. They can also even make a comparatively mediocre display, like an old CGA (color/graphics adapter) monitor, look much crisper and clearer than it actually is. These optical filters absorb unwanted light from the environment, preventing much of it from being reflected at you in the form of glare. The filtering effect on the screen image itself means that you probably need to turn up the contrast and brightness controls to higher levels than are required without a filter. In theory, that may slightly reduce the life of your monitor screen, but a few hundred dollars to replace hardware is a small price to pay to prevent damaging priceless and irreplaceable eyes.

When buying a filter, consider quality *before* price. A good filter should enhance the clarity of screen images, for example making text letters crisper and better defined against their backgrounds. Colors should be more distinctive and separated also. If you take seriously the warnings about low frequency radiation from VDTs, you will probably want a mesh screen that claims to protect against radiation as well as reduce glare. Whatever filter you select, make sure it fits properly for your make, model, and size of monitor so that it covers all the screen area without intruding into the actual display. They are normally fastened into place by adhesive Velcro pads or strips. Some can be molded with the fingers to fit snugly over a monitor with a curved front.

## Clean Screens

Remember to keep both the filter and screen clean, or they will soon attract a layer of dust and other environmental pollutants. Washing instructions vary between types and makes of filters. Some need just a light rinse with water; others require special washing solutions.

The screen itself should be wiped frequently, usually very sparingly with *lightly* soaped warm water followed by rinsing and wiping with a clean, nonscratching cloth. You can get special towelettes to do the job that are suitable for normal and coated surfaces. Some contain antistatic solutions that reduce dust buildup.

Whatever method you use to clean the CRT screen and antiglare filter, use a clean moistened cloth first and a clean dry one second. The other way round, you greatly increase the risk of scratching the screen or filter, which will just add to the problem of unwanted reflections. Rub lightly over the surface and frequently change the area of cloth being used as it becomes dirty. If you do scratch the screen—which may have a plastic surface much softer than glass—you may aggravate glare and other eyestrain problems, as well as face surprisingly big bills to get it professionally restored.

## Upgrade or Tune Hardware and Software

If you have an old monitor, it may fall well below current glare-resistant standards—and the clarity of image fades away as a monitor ages, so consider a replacement. Think also about upgrading, for example from a CGA standard monitor to the much better definition EGA (enhanced graphics adapter) and VGA (video graphics array) standards. However, you may get dramatic improvements in clarity and degree of eyestrain just by fine-tuning the settings of both the monitor controls and the software that generates the images.

Most programs offer options for monitor settings when you first install them, and you should follow these instructions carefully to ensure that you are getting the quality of picture that your software is capable of delivering. With many word processors, for example, you have a considerable range of color choices for both the text and the screen background against which the text is read, as well as a choice of text formats. By experimenting, you may achieve a dramatic improvement. For example, your eyestrain may be reduced considerably by having the font style and size of display that you use most frequently in a shade of yellow against a blue background. Or white on green may be the best combination for you and your equipment. You will not know unless you try, so a trip into the set-up options table can prove very worthwhile.

Screen colors do not seem to be particularly significant for most people, although individual colors and variations do affect some of us. The effects may be emotional—the colors are disagreeable to us and may cause stress subliminally.

## A Rare Phenomenon

A few people are susceptible to what is called the McCullough effect. When we look at green text letters displayed against a dark background for long periods, we see an afterimage in which any white letters or objects have a pink edge to them, or seem to be displayed against a pink background.

This can be frightening the first time you experience it and may persist for days, even weeks, before fading. However, it is a rare phenomenon, so do not let it put you off VDTs that have restful green screens with clear white text. If you are not susceptible to the McCullough effect, you may find such VDTs more comfortable to use for tasks such as word processing or programming than color displays.

Amber-colored displays have done well in comparative tests for comfortable reading, so they are worth considering.

## The Flicker Problem

Some monitors have an inherent tendency to flicker, or develop this characteristic with voltage fluctuations as they get hotter after prolonged use, or flicker when displaying particular software programs. This can be a cause of eyestrain, headaches, nausea, fatigue, and stress. All screens flicker—their displays are "refreshed" about 60 times a second by streams of electrons bombarding the surface. If the monitor is not set up correctly, or if it has deteriorated with age, flickering can reach distressing levels.

Flicker tends to be a problem directly proportional to how much you pay for your hardware. The top-of-the-line VGA and Super VGA and the IBM 8514 standard monitors show great progress in reducing flicker. If you are doing intensive desktop publishing or CAD work in which color is not required, consider also a high-quality "paper white" monitor. The expense may well be worth it, for your eyes' sake.

You can also tackle the flicker problem through the board or card in your computer that controls the video display. The fault may lie there, or you may be able to get a much better image on a monitor by upgrading the card. For example, Genoa Systems introduced the first Super VGA card specifically tackling the flicker problem by refreshing the screen image more frequently than the usual 60 frames per second.

## Focusing Problems

Some early research findings indicate that VDT screens may cause a rapid deterioration in the ability of the eyes to focus. This happens naturally with age, but such problems have been reported also among young people using computers. The symptoms include blurring when you change focus, e.g., by looking from the screen to distant objects through a window and back again.

If you experience such difficulties, do not delay in having your eyes tested and getting professional advice. You should also have your eyes tested regularly—at least once a year—if you do a lot of computer work, and tell your ophthalmologist that you use a VDT. But do not automatically blame vision problems on computer work, although there is mounting evidence that VDTs both cause and aggravate a wide range of ocular conditions.

There are various ways to use software programs to increase clarity and reduce eyestrain from a computer screen. A screen dump showing the Eye Relief word processing program's large, clear type is shown in Figure 2. It is particularly useful with laptops. You can also increase the legibility of any word processor simply by displaying the text with double, instead of single, spacing between the lines.

## Eyeglasses

Do not assume that the eyeglasses you wear normally, or for special close work or reading, are suitable for use with a computer monitor. Reading glasses, bifocals, and trifocals can all cause problems at the keyboard when you are sitting in an ergonomically correct position and at least two feet from the computer screen.

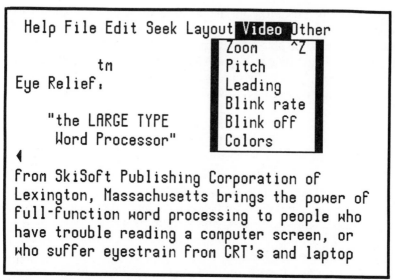

Figure   2. The large, clear type of the Eye Relief word
           processing program.

You may need to change your habits as well as your glasses, perhaps moving printed material farther away into the same plane of focus as the monitor screen. You can hold papers in this position on a special adjustable stand sold for the purpose or with the document clips that go on the side of the monitor. (A health warning here on your computer's behalf! Don't use metal document holders with magnets to hold the papers in position. If the magnets come near your disks, they could well scramble your files.)

You may need glasses just for computing, or an additional pair of bifocals that enables you to focus on the monitor screen, rather than at a normal reading distance. Consider progressive trifocals, which combine in one pair of lenses a lower area to focus at reading distance, a middle range for the monitor, and an upper area for normal distance viewing.

Opinion among opticians varies considerably over the merits of tinting spectacles for computer work and to help combat strain from fluorescent lights. If you have persistent problems, try tinting. Some yellow tints are claimed to reduce glare and help focus. Gray tints are claimed to be restful.

But first, if glare from the monitor is bad enough to make you consider wearing variants of sunglasses indoors, you should go back a few pages and first try our tips to fix the environmental problems. Get your computer workplace to conform to your needs, don't force yourself to adapt to it.

---

# Quick Fix #12

You may suspect overhead fluorescent lights are causing your problems. In many offices they cannot be switched off without plunging the whole room—even the whole floor—into darkness. Temporarily tape heavy-duty black plastic garbage bags over the lights to see if that makes an improvement. If it does, call maintenance or an electrician to selectively switch off the lights affecting your work area, or remove the tubes. Maintain satisfactory illumination levels for paperwork with independent workstation lighting.

---

## Emotional Impact of Eyestrain

Whether your eyes are tense or relaxed can have a profound effect on your psychological and emotional well being. Remember, eyes are the softest, most vulnerable part of the body that is exposed to the external world. They are your most sensitive interface with your environment, so nurture them carefully.

You abuse your eyes if you allow them to gaze fixedly at the harsh images on the computer display. Just like your body, they become overstressed and need regular exercise and rest. Allow them to relax and exercise, to look out of the window, or perhaps rest occasionally on a favorite picture or vase of flowers.

## Exercise Your Eyes to Protect Your Vision

All movements of the eyes, as well as how they adjust to distance and light, are controlled by muscles. Although much smaller than those of your back and neck, these muscles can get just as tight and frozen. They can contribute, without your realizing it, to your shoulder and neck tension and headaches.

Consequently, it is important for you to exercise them regularly, just like other muscles that are affected by your work.

In fact, because the eyes are the most overworked part of the computer operator's body, they need special exercise attention to keep them fit and to counteract the negative consequences of our work.

Biologically, eyes are designed to scan constantly at varying distances, both in front of you at the objects of your attention and peripherally to alert you to possible threats from the sides. When reading print—or a monitor display—for hours on end, the eyes are being trained to see a limited two-dimensional area in front of you, not the wider three-dimensional view that is natural to them and for which they were designed.

The eyes get locked into this unnatural two-dimensional pattern. So you will find it very helpful to relax your eyes and intentionally see three-dimensionally when you are not working. In doing this, you will become pleasantly relaxed as your eyes begin to let go of their computer-programmed pattern and see normally again.

## Quick Fix #13

Learn to see again like a natural animal when you are walking. Consciously relax your eyes and let them wander, especially to the sides and up and down. Allow them to linger on pleasing shapes, colors, and textures. For example, when you see a tree, allow your eyes to roam from the base up to the top branches. Give your eyes a holiday from the fixed stare of computer work.

There are also several ways that you can relax and exercise your eyes during your work time at the computer. Become conscious of the feeling of weight in your eyes when they are tense, and how much more comfortable and lighter they feel when you relax them.

One way to achieve this eye relaxation is to imagine that your eyes are clenched and then consciously loosen them. Another is to soften your focus and reach out three-dimensionally to the farthest point you can see.

While computing, do not allow your head to lean forward and your eyes to bug out to see what is on the screen. Relax, with your head balanced vertically on your shoulders, and allow the screen images to float toward you.

Many people eventually need to wear eyeglasses, but some who have been coached in vision exercise and therapy have reported impressive improvements to the point where they can see clearly again without glasses. If you are interested in getting professional vision therapy, try seeing a behavioral optometrist. These optometrists, who prescribe glasses and measure eye performance, generally tend to be more favorably disposed to this holistic methodology than ophthalmologists—the eye doctors and surgeons.

Listed below are exercises that all take less than a minute, but which can do a great deal to help your eyes remain healthy and cope with the stress of computing.

These exercises may also help to ease headaches. Some you may find difficult or uncomfortable at first. Concentrate on the others, and then return to the difficult ones later as you learn better how to relax and exercise your eyes.

1. Focus your eyes as far away as you can see, on the horizon if that is in view.
2. Soften your visual focus and scan the environment of your office or room. Linger while in this soft-focus mode on the shapes, outlines, and colors that you see.
3. Alternate quickly between looking at a distant object and a close one. Do this several times, and use your peripheral vision as well. This is a valuable exercise in itself and a good warm-up for the next exercise.
4. While holding your head still, visually trace an infinity pattern—a horizontal figure 8 ($\infty$)—first in one direction and then in the other. Try to move your eyes in as large a pattern as you can.
5. Intentionally unfocus your eyes for a short period of time. Feel the relaxation this causes in the muscles of your upper cheeks and above the eyes.

6. With your fingertips, massage the muscles above and below your eyes.
7. Raise and lower your eyebrows four times in an action similar to shrugging your shoulders. Move them as high and as low as you can. This will relax the facial muscles around the eyes that can become very tense as you read.
8. Trace diagonals with your eyes. Without moving your head, look at the upper left corner of your visual field and then move your eyes to the lower right corner. Move back up to your starting point. Do this for the other diagonal as well.
9. Rub your hands together vigorously so that your palms become warm. Then press the fleshy part of your palms against your closed eyelids. Feel the warmth spread into your eyes. This is a good final exercise.

You can also relax your eyes and ease the muscles around them by lying down with a soft, damp cloth over them.

Diet and emotional stress can also have an impact on the health of your eyes.

# 3

# *The Truth About Headaches—and What You Can Do to Stop Them*

Almost everybody suffers from headaches at one time or another, and computer users are even more disposed to them than the average person.

A National Institutes of Health survey of more than 10,000 Americans found that 95 percent of women and 90 percent of men had at least one headache in the previous year. Forty-five million Americans every year get headaches so severe they seek treatment. The situation is similar in other developed countries.

Over 150 million Americans annually suffer at least one severe headache, and much working time is lost due to headaches. General physicians alone are consulted nearly 20 million times a year for headaches and prescribe some 60 million analgesic medications to ease head pain. Headache sufferers consume 40 million pounds of aspirin annually, plus lots of other medications, in their search for relief.

So headaches are big business. Americans probably spend over a billion dollars a year trying to stop pain in their head. Most of that goes for very profitable drugs and highly promoted "cures," most of which really do very little, if anything, to help headache sufferers get long-term relief. In fact, there is no drug that will *cure* headache—yet billions of dollars are pumped into advertising that claims many medicines will do just that.

Of course, there are "painkillers" that may give temporary relief, but their habitual use by headache sufferers can be dangerous. It is extraordinary that we ban cigarette advertising from television but do comparatively little to alert the public to the potential dangers of proprietary painkillers, most of which are used—and abused—by headache sufferers, including millions of computer users.

According to the National Center for Health Statistics, in nearly three-quarters of the visits headache sufferers make to American physicians, the doctors prescribe analgesic medications. But the 60 million such prescriptions for headaches written every year are having no long-term beneficial effect on the incidence of head pain.

So millions of people each year have their lives disrupted by headaches, yet there is enormous ignorance about the causes, the treatments, and the ways to prevent this distressing health problem. But we have very good news for you. Out of all this confusion and commercial exploitation comes the fundamental truth that there are solutions to most headache problems—including those suffered by computer users. The truth is that nearly all headaches can be prevented or cured without pills by actions we can take ourselves.

## Nearly All Headaches Can Be Prevented or Cured

Muscle tension causes the majority of headaches, with dilation of the cranial arteries being responsible for many migraine attacks, the most serious form of headache pain. We can do much ourselves, by modifying our work and life-styles, and by proper diet, exercise, breathing, and posture, to control the causes of most headaches.

Headaches often are linked directly to emotional states, principally feelings of fear, anger, and frustration that we are trying to suppress. Everybody—and we mean *everybody*—has natural feelings or emotions which society has taught us to suppress. But these basic emotions do not go away. We retain them subconsciously and express them through muscle tension and muscle contraction. In other words, we really do get "uptight"!

Emotional states are expressed particularly in the soft tissues of the body—most of which are muscle tissue. When these muscles are held contracted over long periods, they tend to become locked. When this occurs in the shoulder, neck, and head region—as often happens to computer users—a headache often results.

It is believed that animals do not suffer from the human type of headache. Nor did prehistoric man: nor do many primitive people still living naturally in remote parts of the world. Most headaches are a direct consequence of our fast-paced twentieth-century life-style, particularly computing work styles that do not pay due regard to health considerations.

At the Neurologic Center for Headache and Pain in La Jolla, California, the director, Dr. David Hubbard, and his team concentrate on head pain.

Over a hundred patients a week go to the La Jolla center, most of them referred by doctors who have been unable to help them. They seek out Dr. Hubbard because chronic recurring headaches are utterly miserable and can destroy the quality of life.

Most chronic recurring head pain defies conventional diagnosis and treatment, yet the headache center is achieving a nearly 87 percent success rate with patients who complete the treatment procedure there, the highest documented success rate in treating headache anywhere. Dr. Hubbard and his colleagues are demonstrating, without any shadow of doubt, that headache can be cured by the patients themselves when they learn to control their fears, their anger, and the stress in their lives.

According to Dr. Hubbard and his staff, of the thousands of patients who have walked into their consulting rooms, not one really knew the cause of his or her recurring head pain. That is in part because many of the general physicians they previously consulted are woefully ignorant about headache and tend not to spend much time on such a complaint, which is difficult to treat and rarely life-threatening.

In 93 percent of visits to a doctor for problems relating to headache, the consultation lasts fifteen minutes or less. But a new patient's first appointment at the headache center is always scheduled for ninety minutes. Dr. Hubbard says that most of that first consultation is spent helping the patient to separate headache fact from fantasy. The ignorance is mainly a consequence of the pharmaceutical companies and other vested interests' disseminating information to promote their products and services that is, at best, misleading, and often downright false.

There *is* high-quality, accurate, and up-to-date information about headaches. But it is largely confined to very technical textbooks and learned journals that only specialists read and can comprehend. The scientific community knows a great deal about headaches but does not communicate that information so that ordinary intelligent people can benefit from their knowledge. A notable exception is the National Headache Foundation, which offers members much helpful information. The foundation is located at 5252 N. Western Avenue, Chicago, IL 60625. You can call the foundation toll-free at 1-800-523-8858 in Illinois, or 1-800-843-2256 from other states.

## Essential Headache Facts

Before we get into the details of what you as a computer user need to know about the safe, practical ways to prevent or ease the types of headaches you are likely to encounter, let's look at some basic facts about headaches. They will prepare you to approach head pain from a more informed viewpoint and so be well on the way to achieving a permanent solution.

### Fact 1

Continuing to take aspirin, or any other painkillers promoted as headache "cures," is not only a waste of time but can actually make your headache worse and cause other health problems. There are *no* medications that have been proven to cure chronic headaches.

### Fact 2

Many medical tests, including the most expensive, are not necessary or really helpful in diagnosing the cause of most head pain. The main exceptions are cases where there is trauma resulting from physical damage (as in an accident) and brain tumors.

### Fact 3

There are only two causes for virtually all headaches—muscle tension and blood vessel constriction/dilation. These are usually controllable, so effective cures are possible, even in many very severe cases.

### Fact 4

The muscle tension and vascular constriction that cause headache for the most part result directly from either emotional triggers or the unnecessary physical stresses caused by poor posture combined with bad work habits. There is substantial evidence that the common cause of both muscle tension and vascular change is suppressed emotional feelings. However, to deal with their problems effectively, computer users in particular must also take into consideration the stress and injury caused by the mechanical misuse of their bodies.

## Posture and Pain at the Keyboard

Your working posture at the keyboard, your diet, and the emotional pressures created by your work situation are among the major factors to consider in reducing the tension that leads to headaches.

Your hardware and software may also play a specific role, with a bad screen display a frequent culprit. Inferior displays may create constant tension and stress in your eyes, one of the chief contributors to headache in computer users. Or your equipment may force you to adopt a stressful position for extensive periods. For example, you may find yourself twisted in your chair with your head at a stressed, uncomfortable angle to overcome the effects of glare on the screen from an overhead light or the sun shining through a window. Such tensioning of muscles and joints can create head pain.

## Types of Headaches

Following are discussions of various types of common headaches, symptoms, and some possible remedies.

## Tension Headaches

Most headaches—probably nine out of ten—are caused by muscle contraction. There is usually a steady pain, perhaps accompanied by a feeling of tightness in the scalp. The pain is usually generalized in the head area, and sometimes radiates down the neck. It is rarely localized. You minimize the risk of such headache by following our advice on exercise and posture.

Unfortunately, we can't suggest one Quick Fix to cure all the headaches that computer users experience. You must be prepared to devote some effort to achieving a correct sitting posture, changing your computing position regularly, taking frequent breaks, and doing the appropriate exercises.

Many tension headaches are caused by overworking the trapezius muscles—running from your shoulders toward the back of your head—and the splenius muscles of the neck, both of which are linked to the base of your skull. These muscles can become very contracted as a result of emotional tension or holding your head forward in an unnatural position over the keyboard for long periods. General work stress and adverse environmental factors greatly increase the tension.

We become particularly vulnerable to tension headaches after a long period of sustained computer work. Learn to recognize when you are approaching the danger time and stop computing. Always try to stretch and relax these muscles periodically by using the shoulder and neck exercises in Chapter 5. Improve your work posture by using the methods in Chapter 1.

## Vascular Headaches

Vascular headaches include migraines and are the second most common form of head pain. They are caused by constriction and expansion of the blood vessels, so a pulsing, throbbing sensation is often present.

In contrast to tension headaches, the cluster form of vascular headaches is characterized by pain focused on one place, usually above, behind, or near one eye. The onset of pain may be associated with chemical stressors, including foods, drinks, and environmental pollutants.

### Sinus Headaches

Sinus headaches, caused by inflamed mucous membranes, are the least common type. Painkillers may ease discomfort in the areas of the forehead, nose, and cheeks, but the cause of the pain will usually not go away without appropriate treatment.

### Infection and Disease

A very small proportion of headaches are caused by infections, diseases, tumors, or other specific medical conditions. Although responsible for less than one in a hundred headaches, such potentially serious causes should be checked out by a medical specialist in any case of recurring headaches, or one that is sudden, very severe, or results in loss of consciousness, vomiting, or other similar disturbing symptoms.

## Reduce Stress

There is no pain more universal than headaches, yet also none so preventable and treatable simply by reducing the stress in your life. In addition to the specific guidelines for reducing stress in computer work found in Chapter 8, the National Headache Foundation recommends the following stress reducers.

- Get up fifteen minutes earlier in the morning. The inevitable morning mishaps will be less stressful.
- Prepare for the morning the evening before. Set up the breakfast table, make lunches, put out the clothes you plan to wear.
- Don't rely on your memory. Write down things like appointment times, when to pick up the laundry, when library books are due.
- Make duplicates of all keys. Bury a house key in a secret spot in the garden and carry a duplicate car key in your wallet, apart from your key ring.
- Be prepared to wait. A paperback can make a wait in a post office line much less unpleasant.

- Allow fifteen minutes of extra time to get to appointments.
- Unplug your phone if you want to take a long bath, meditate, sleep, or read without interruption.
- Get enough sleep.
- Organize your home and work space so that you always know exactly where things are.
- Don't forget to take a lunch break. Try to get away from your desk or work area in body and mind, even if it's just for fifteen or twenty minutes.

The National Headache Foundation says that events causing emotional stress are among the most frequent precipitating factors in migraine attacks. The mental fatigue so often experienced by computer users can combine with muscle tension to trigger a migraine attack.

These and other conditions involving headache respond well to the stress and tension reduction exercises in Chapter 5.

## Be a "Headache Detective" (Discover the Causes)

Linking symptoms to their cause in the search for solutions to head pain may require considerable detective work. For example, headaches may occur when you try to relax, rather than, as would seem most likely, at the peak of your stress and tension. This is because your blood vessels, after being constricted because of the tension, dilate when you relax and so trigger a headache. Consequently, this type of headache often occurs on weekends, after you think you are free from the consequences of a stressful workweek.

If you suffer from this type of headache, you may need to both reduce the continual intensity of stress at work and introduce a transition period from these very tense work phases to your periods of complete relaxation. Remember also that our life-styles often result in leisure periods, such as weekends, which introduce other forms of stress. Any change, especially a rapid one, can be a stressor that triggers a headache when the tension pattern has already built up. Business travel, for example, involves stresses and changes that may easily trigger headaches.

You may be triggering headaches by such unconscious habits as holding your breath, clenching your jaw, or adopting a fixed staring position when concentrating for long periods on your computing activity. All of these patterns are very common in almost all headache situations. Ask family, friends, or colleagues to observe you at work and draw your attention to any such possible headache triggers.

Relief in some cases can be achieved by massaging your jaw, neck, and scalp muscles. A gently oscillating battery-powered massager can loosen stiff muscles, but nothing beats human fingers.

Tension patterns start young. Children particularly tend to tense up their muscles when playing computer games—and children, as well as adults, suffer from headaches. So observe your children at the computer, or when playing Nintendo games, and intervene with corrective suggestions and more frequent breaks to prevent potential headache patterns from developing.

You may notice that your children are developing breath-holding habits when concentrating at the computer, on video games, or when studying. Slouching and other bad sitting postures also may develop at an early age and become lifelong habits. Rather than just telling children to sit up straight, explain to them why correct posture is important. You will give your children lifelong benefits.

## Environmental Triggers

Many stressors in your computing environment can trigger headaches. When the National Headache Foundation surveyed over 3,000 migraine sufferers, nearly a third identified smoking as a stimulus for their attacks. If you are working in a smoky atmosphere, the contaminated air may cause changes in the biological makeup of your blood and in the blood vessels, causing headaches when the vessels distend or contract.

Noise and light are two other important environmental stress factors. Be particularly careful if you are a headache sufferer of exposure to slowly flickering light, which may come from the fluorescent lamps in your workplace or from your monitor screen.

Full-spectrum fluorescent lights in the room are much calmer for the eyes and have been shown to have a positive psychological effect compared to other artificial lighting. Seek permanent solutions to eliminate lighting problems. You may get some temporary relief at the terminal, especially if the flickering light is bright, from wearing

Polaroid glasses or having a polarizing filter in front of the screen of a troublesome VDT. But excessive flickering or other instability of the image indicates either an inferior monitor or one due for replacement. Never tolerate such faults, because they can be harmful.

Some migraine sufferers experience attacks when they breathe in dry air containing a high proportion of electrically charged dust particles—the kind of conditions that frequently arise in a computing environment. You may obtain considerable relief by positioning a humidifier near you, perhaps a small one with an outlet that can be controlled so that the moist air is directed at you, not at the hardware.

Strong smells may trigger a migraine attack in susceptible people. When new, some computer hardware can emit a strong plastic chemical odor as the equipment heats up. This condition should not persist and may be alleviated by good ventilation.

---

℞

# Quick Fix #14

Clean out the inside of a PC case frequently to remove dust, which can smell as the electronic components heat up. You may ease some of your headache and allergy problems—and protect your hardware at the same time, because many computer failures are caused by the overheating of dirty equipment.

---

It is a myth that computer equipment must be kept in a very dry environment. Your hardware may be more at risk from the buildup of static electricity in exceptionally dry conditions than from moisture in the air when humidity levels are comfortable for human operators.

Older equipment in particular may smell because of a buildup of dust particles settling onto hot electronic components. It requires no technical skill to remove the cover from a PC and gently blow or vacuum away the buildup of dust every year as preventive medicine for both your system and yourself. You should do this more frequently if working in a very dusty or dry environment. If you use a vacuum, be careful not to dislodge or disturb sensitive components or get the electric motor of the vacuum so close that the magnetic fields it generates damage your equipment or data files.

A particular problem is the odor emitted by some kinds of synthetic carpet found in many offices. Even the staff at the Environmental Protection Agency experienced this in a celebrated case of potentially hazardous office conditions. Get an EPA or other qualified investigator to check if you think the carpets, air conditioning, or other sources of odors or fumes are triggering headaches or causing other health problems.

Varying weather conditions, including barometric pressure, can cause or aggravate headache problems. So even if you are an ardent laptop user, it may not be wise to compute intensively during or immediately after flights if you are susceptible to headaches.

## Dietary Triggers

Unless you have severe food allergy susceptibility, by following our dietary recommendations in Chapter 6, you should not have cause to blame your food for any headaches you suffer. But if you eat irregularly, particularly junk food or food and drink that contain additives or have been aged or fermented, you may well aggravate your headache problem.

Migraine attacks and headaches in general may be triggered by chocolate, cheese, alcohol, fried foods, tenderizers, monosodium glutamate, and nitrates or nitrites in processed foods.

Headaches that you attribute to the computer may well stem from some particular allergen in your diet to which you are sensitive or from something in your environment that provokes an allergic reaction. These can be identified by process of elimination, or if this proves ineffective, by medical tests.

The best diets for headache sufferers in particular—and all computer users in general—contain fresh, natural foods.

# 4

# *Repetitive Stress Injury*

Carpal tunnel syndrome (CTS) is perhaps the most specific and most publicized condition caused by the repetitive stress of hand and wrist actions repeated frequently over a long period. CTS belongs to a category of injuries called cumulative trauma disorders that accounts for about half of the confirmed work-related injuries in the United States.

As we will see later, repetitive stress injuries (RSIs) are a much bigger—and growing—problem than official statistics, policies, or legislation reflect. Already they cause more than 16 million lost workdays each year. The total is much greater if you include professionals and self-employed people who tend to be heavy computer users but whose health problems are not well documented. Inevitably, as computer use extends throughout our society, RSI problems will increase.

CTS is the health problem that can be, at this stage of human experience with keyboards and with the limited research into the subject, most confidently blamed on improper computer use. The symptoms are abnormal pain, numbness, weakness, and burning or tingling sensations in the fingers and hands, sometimes extending to the elbows. You may first experience these discomforts at night, not necessarily while working.

CTS results from compression of the median nerve in the carpal tunnel, a small tunnel located in the wrist just below the thumb. In extreme cases, the condition becomes chronic and results in partial paralysis of the hand and deterioration of the large muscle at the base of the thumb (thenarus).

---

℞

# Quick Fix #15

Remember the two words "finger flow" whenever you work at the keyboard. A prime cause of carpal tunnel syndrome and other RSI problems in the hand, wrist, and arm is keyboarding with a sharp upward angle to the wrist. If your fingers when they are hitting the keys are higher than your wrists then you are on the road to pain.

Imagine your thoughts flowing down from your brain through your neck, shoulders, arms, wrists, and fingers to reach the computer through your fingertips as they stroke the keys. Always sit and work so that this flow is as smooth and unimpeded as possible. Angling your hands and fingers upward from the wrist creates an obvious interruption to the flow. You must adopt the correct posture to achieve the proper coordination and integration of body function that best protects us against computer-related, repetitive stress injuries.

---

This nerve compression results when the open space inside the carpal tunnel becomes constricted so that pressure is put directly on the median nerve. Computer users are vulnerable to localized inflammation or swelling of the tissues in this area because keyboards, mice, and trackballs encourage us to have bad working habits and to misuse the delicate structures of the arm, wrist, and hand.

The microtrauma that results from this misuse is called *repetitive stress injury* or *cumulative trauma disorder,* which is the accumulation of microinjuries.

The surgical method of dealing with this problem is called a *carpal tunnel release,* a freeing of the ligaments that hold the carpal tunnel in a position that irritates the median nerve. This may seem to be a logical and effective way to restore normal nerve function. However, for the serious computer user it may be an expensive and uncomfortable experience that obtains only limited and temporary relief.

If medical and surgical treatment attempts only to correct the symptoms, the actual cause of the problem will remain and the injury will be repeated. Much better than resorting to the knife is identifying bad work habits and treating them as well as the painful condition, preferably in good time to prevent chronic problems from occurring. How workers interface with their computers is both the cause of and the solution to most repetitive stress injuries.

## Myths and Misconceptions

Myths and misconceptions about repetitive stress injury and carpal tunnel syndrome abound. The business community and federal and state government agencies still tend to dismiss it as not having great significance. The few publicized cases usually occur when a group of workers in a particular company or industry are successful in getting CTS both diagnosed and recognized as a consequence of computer work.

Then skeptics claim that there has been a form of epidemic hysteria, in which psychological factors in the group of workers are transferred into shared physical symptoms. The outbreak also may be blamed on "compensationitis," with the suggestion that the computer workers are faking or aggravating their pain to seek financial compensation.

Neither of these nonsenses is a credible explanation of the quantity and variety of outbreaks of RSI among computer users and other workers all over the world. Although accurate information and statistics on RSIs are woefully inadequate in the United States and most of Europe, an unusual combination of circumstances cleared up many of the myths and misconceptions years ago in Australia.

## Lessons From Down Under

Repetitive stress injuries became prominent in Australia in the mid-1980s. RSIs were so little recognized in other parts of the world at that time that the condition was known as "kangaroo paw" and regarded by many as a purely Australian phenomenon.

Australia is blessed with enlightened workers compensation legislation and a legal system that is not as adversarial as the one in the United States. These factors have made it far easier for the Australian business community, unions, medical profession, and politicians to recognize and tackle the reality that computers are hurting people. In particular, it is far, far easier in Australia for a worker to establish that microtrauma caused by work has created a medical problem. In the United States, we still classify RSI as a disease rather than an injury. Linking a disease and the responsibility for it to employment can take years of protracted, expensive testing and litigation. It is much easier to pursue a claim successfully in the United States if you suffer a traumatic injury—like falling down and breaking your leg because the floor is wet—than if you are disabled because the computing workstation is defective and injures you more slowly and subtly.

The Australians confronted the problem of repetitive stress microtrauma by simply classifying all occupational medical problems stemming from overuse of body functions as repetition strain injury. This is a broad classification that everybody can understand, and it makes the problem easily identifiable. In contrast, in the United States and Europe we have cluttered and confused the issue by applying many different labels to RSI, which has made identification much more difficult.

In the United States, the evidence required to confirm a diagnosis of RSI may be onerous and expensive to obtain. There are actually very powerful forces at work in this country to suppress the identification and quantification of RSI.

Even when substantial evidence is assembled, employers, insurers, and lawyers can prevent or delay confirmation of RSI and the consequent financial settlement of a disability or liability claim. Government agencies are as bad in this respect as the commercial sector. Even at the Social Security Administration headquarters near Baltimore, computer operators diagnosed with RSI have waited years while their cases were documented and evaluated. Some even had carpal tunnel surgery while they were waiting.

Since the 1970s the U.S. Postal Service has resisted accepting that keyboard operation of letter sorting machines causes RSI. There is strong evidence that many of the 50,000 letter sorting machine operators have RSI. The American Postal Workers Union testified to Congress that 30 percent of operators had been diagnosed with CTS or tendonitis, with 20 percent suffering so much pain that surgery was prescribed.

So United States government statistics do not even reflect the seriousness of RSI among its own employees, let alone give any reliable indication of the extent of the problem among computer operators in the business community. The Reagan administration's cutbacks to the Occupational Health and Safety Administration (OSHA) made it even more difficult during the 1980s to assemble the information we now so desperately need. In contrast, the Australian government immediately set up a task force on RSI and has made great progress in tackling this problem.

## The Female Factor

An important lesson we can learn from the Australians is that there is ample proof that RSI is a genuine physical malady, not a psychological hysteria phenomenon to which female workers are particularly susceptible.

The hysteria theory has been fueled by sexist interpretations of the fact that RSI appears to affect women two to five times more frequently than men. The Australians found simple explanations for this that have largely been overlooked here in the United States. Women predominate overwhelmingly in the type of repetitive keyboard computer work that most often leads to RSI. Women also tend to be shorter than men—both in overall height and in the length of their lower arms. Desks and other workstations are built to standard dimensions that make it much more likely that a man rather than a woman will operate a keyboard with an ergonomically satisfactory posture.

Women working at standard-height desks are almost always forced into a posture that imposes stress on that critical wrist area where the median nerve enters the carpal tunnel. Consequently, they are far more likely to injure the nerve fibers responsible for both movement and feeling. The almost inevitable consequences are pain and disablement.

The hysteria and compensationitis theories also take a knock from the incontrovertible evidence that RSI problems have been recorded at times and in places where neither the influence of other people nor the prospect of compensation played any role. RSI is not confined to computer operators working for deep-pocket big companies. It is also commonly observed among self-employed people—musicians, for example—who have very little to gain from seeking compensation for injury and much to lose if they cannot pursue their professions.

## Serious Economic Consequences

Although the few reliable statistics available do not reflect the rapidly increasing incidence of RSI, they do give an indication of the extent and cost of the problem. In 1984, the American Academy of Orthopedic Surgeons conducted a study that indicated that the direct costs for all musculoskeletal injuries were in excess of $22 billion.

International studies indicate that about a third of all injuries to workers involve the hand and upper extremity, with microtrauma resulting from repetitive stress injury steadily increasing both this proportion and the overall numbers.

## Getting Treatment That Works

The first step in getting effective treatment if you suspect you have RSI problems is to find a medical or chiropractic doctor who is well-informed on the holistic correction of this problem. The wrong advice can trap you in a frustrating, expensive, and ineffective cycle of consultations, medications, steroid injections, and surgical procedures.

Agreeing to even the most common of the surgical "solutions" is a step not to be taken lightly. The carpal tunnel release surgical procedure requires at least the cutting of the flexor retinaculum of the wrist. Further cutting and surgical work may be required, depending on the severity of the case. Some patients undergo extensive cleaning out of inflamed tissues before the pressure on the median nerve is reduced sufficiently for normal nerve function to be restored. Surgery is usually followed by a considerable period of hand and wrist immobility—which in itself can cause further physical and psychological problems. It is very easy to become so preoccupied with your RSI condition that you become severely depressed, perceive the symptoms to be worse than they actually may be, and dwell on the prospect of permanent disability.

However, researchers have found that full, informed cooperation between doctors and therapists experienced with RSI and motivated computer-user victims can *reduce the need for medical consultation by over two thirds* within as little as three months.

## Tackle the Causes, Not the Symptoms

Initial treatment efforts must pay due consideration to the individual circumstances of the patient and the patient's job, not just respond to the symptoms and the diagnosis in isolation. Modification of work and other activities that localize stress to a particular body part will frequently result in a successful outcome without surgery.

Three major work factors must be dealt with:

1. *Posture* is the most important consideration. How you sit at the computer determines how efficiently—or inefficiently—you use your joints, muscles, and body in general.

2. *Repetition* is also a major factor. The more repetitive the task is, the more rapid and frequent are the muscular contractions necessary to carry it out. Consequently, the likelihood of RSI from overuse increases. A task requiring a certain amount of muscle effort may present no risk at all until it is repeated over prolonged periods.

3. *Fatigue* is critical also. Often work style and other pressures force us to continue computing in a fatigued state. Your body works less efficiently and becomes more prone to injury at such times.

## Regulations Can Be Effective and Inexpensive

There is an urgent need to establish standards and regulations for repetitive computer work. When coupled with simple training, exercise, and other programs, they need not impose the cost burdens that the business community seems to fear so much—and the results can be impressive. Take the example of Ethicon, Inc.

*The Journal of Hand Surgery* published a paper in September 1987 titled "Cumulative trauma disorder controls: The ergonomics program at Ethicon, Inc." by George Lutz, M.D., and Terri Hansford, R.P.T. It describes how, in 1978, the medical staff of Ethicon were faced with an increased incidence of inflammatory and nerve entrapment syndromes that occurred primarily at the wrist and hand. These problems served as the impetus for the development of an ergonomics program for the control of cumulative trauma disorders.

℞

# Quick Fix #16

Establish your own task force to learn how exposed you or your computer operators are to RSI. Run through this checklist and, if you identify problems, get them fixed—quickly!

- Can you adjust your table, desk, chair, and monitor easily?
- Are they adjusted correctly for the user?
- Is there a natural flow of thought and motion, particularly down through arms and fingers so that wrists are not angled upward or used in isolation from the arm and shoulder?
- Are wrists or forearms being stressed by resting on the edge of the table or other hard edge? Are wrist rests, even if soft, used incorrectly, putting pressure indirectly on median nerve and isolating finger movement from the wrist and arm?
- Are there repetitive actions that can be reduced or eliminated? Can you create macros or otherwise automate repetitive keyboarding or mouse movement tasks?
- Is it practical and cost-efficient to scan printed data to reduce routine keyboarding?
- Can you institute changes elsewhere in the organization that will reduce your keyboarding work load? Are you keyboarding data or text that someone else has already computerized? If so, can you get an electronic rather than a printed copy of that work so that the keyboarding does not have to be repeated?
- Are operators unduly pressured by monitoring of their performance, incentive programs, or piecework payments so that the risk of overstressing them is increased?
- Are there frequent rest breaks or changes of work activities so that computer operators change their working positions at regular intervals?
- Is workplace clean and uncluttered to reduce stress and ensure that keyboard and mouse can be used comfortably?
- Is there space for documents and other work materials so that they can be used comfortably without conflicting with computing activities?
- Are managers and supervisors aware of computing health hazards and the preventive measures to take?

The company established an ergonomics task force to create a working environment that enhanced productivity by the safe design of the workplace and the promotion of health and wellness. The task force's main objectives were:

1. To intervene in existing ergonomics problems
2. To prevent new ergonomics problems from developing
3. To involve the worker in the ergonomics program

The task force members found that exercise intermittently during the workday had both physiological and psychological benefits for employees. These benefits included:

- Improved posture and breathing
- Improved joint flexibility and muscle extensibility
- Balanced muscle tone
- Improved blood flow
- Reduced risk of inflammation
- Reduced stress

The basic principles and techniques used were consistent in all the participating departments of the company, but the exercises themselves were tailored to the nature of the work performed in each work area.

The RSI problem at Ethicon was reduced by two thirds as a result of this regular and appropriate exercise program.

The lesson is that the company got such good results because the task force established a system to tackle the RSI problems *proactively* rather than *reactively*. The returns extended beyond reduction in RSI rates, reducing also the company's medical costs and significantly improving worker attitude, with all the benefits to the bottom line that implies.

## Keyboards and Mice

Before blaming your keyboard or your mouse or other interface device for RSI pain, you should probably blame yourself. Most of the problems come from our own bad habits, rather than inferior design or functioning of computer hardware.

Resting your wrists on the desk or your arms on the chair is unhealthy because this isolates and weakens mechanical function. When you rest your wrist, you inevitably prevent your fingers from having the proper movement coordination linking them to the rest of your body.

Hand and finger movements—particularly those that are repeated—must be connected to the arms, the shoulders, and the upper back. This is the way we are designed to function. If our hands were attached close to our shoulders, then we would not need to use our entire arms. But we have long arms extending from our shoulders to hands to create a well-designed, integrated mechanical movement pattern in which all the joints, muscles, and tendons are as interdependent as the cogs and wheels of a clock mechanism. If any joint is forced to work in isolation, then it becomes stressed beyond its design and is injured.

Also, the angles created by isolating joints unnaturally can be very injurious. If you lean on your elbows all the time, you isolate hand and wrist movement and create stressful unnatural postures in which the shoulders are held up and the head leans forward.

A particular consequence of continually resting the wrist is that it isolates hand function from the muscles underneath the arm that control this motion and are needed for keyboarding and mouse control. These muscles and tendons need to pull in a straight line, in a movement that coordinates many muscles and joints at the same time. They cannot do that if the wrist and elbow are resting at angles that interfere with smooth, mechanical coordination.

Your fingers should not merely operate the keyboard or mouse, but should work in unison with small movements of the arm and shoulders. One of the worst things you can do is rest your wrists on the edge of a table or some other support and then hit the keys or move the mouse with short, separate movements confined just within the finger and hands. That may seem more comfortable for short periods, but it can be very damaging over a long time.

Most of the muscles that operate the fingers are actually a long way away, in the forearms. The fingers are moved by long tendons, similar to pulley ropes, activated by these muscles in the forearm. When you work with your wrist and hand isolated from your arm, you turn a simple mechanical procedure into a complex and stressful one.

When you rest on your elbow, whether you are at the computer or doing other things like leaning against a bar, the muscles on the leaning side lock into spasm. If it becomes a habit, the muscles become deformed to sustain this unnatural posture. Muscle tension becomes a semipermanent feature of the side of your body you lean on.

The body is designed to move and function as a whole, not to act as a prop. Leaning on your elbow creates muscle contractions that build up to tighten your neck and also affect the shoulder and arm that you are subjecting to these very stressful, imbalanced forces.

Think of the head, arms, legs, hands, back, fingers, and other members as building blocks that support each other and rely on their associates for their own stability. The body's building blocks are designed to function as parts of a single whole unit, just as each of the four wheels on a car works in conjunction with the other three to keep the car balanced and enable it to move forward or change direction in an efficient, coordinated way.

## Headaches and Painful Fingers May Go Together

So do not think of health problems like RSI in isolation, but relate them also to such other symptoms of bad computing habits as headaches. The position of your head, the stresses put upon it, and its ability to move and function efficiently are very much determined by the integration of many other body parts functioning together.

When you isolate your arm and use your wrist and fingers separately, you also lose strength and endurance. The fingers hitting the keys, or grasping the mouse and pressing its buttons, are triggered for each action by instructions from the brain that should travel freely through the body and call into action a whole network of nerves, tendons, muscles, and joints. There is a chemical interaction, the conduction of minute pulses of electrical energy, and physical movement similar to cords passing over pulleys and mechanical joints twisting and turning.

But rest your elbow on the arm of your chair and your wrist on the edge of your desk and manipulate the mouse with cramped, tight, isolated finger movements and you inhibit that complex activity and increase the risk of microtrauma.

We are now seeing a rapid escalation of repetitive stress injury among computer operators using desktop publishing and graphics and computer-aided design programs, which require intensive use of the mouse. Most of their problems come more from the way they use the mouse than from the device itself, but the result is the same—an approaching epidemic of serious injuries from this cause alone.

---

℞

# Quick Fix #17

Pamper your hands and wrists. They work hard, so just like an athlete, allow them to warm up before the full stress of vigorous keyboarding.

If you have pain and soreness, get professional help. A commercial wrist splint may give temporary relief, but it is important to be cautious about the use of wrist splints. OSHA has advised against using them at all. Other knowledgeable specialists advise using them only under very specific conditions and with close supervision. Self-treatment with these devices can be dangerous to your health, even though they are available at every corner drugstore. Wearing splints causes a loss of strength in the wrist and makes the joints more susceptible to injury.

"Contrast baths" of alternating hot and cold may be very beneficial. For painful joints, use an electric heating pad set on low, or a bowl of medium hot water, and an ice or cold pack. Start with 5 minutes of heat, then 7–8 minutes of cold. Repeat three to five times, ending with a long cold session of about 12–15 minutes.

These contrast baths greatly improve circulation in the injured areas, soothing them and promoting healing.

---

## Selecting Hardware to Reduce RSI

Cheap, inferior interface devices are false economies when you think of the risk of RSI from using them repeatedly. Go for good-quality keyboards with a smooth, comfortable action. The keys should be big and ergonomically well laid out. Some layouts very slightly from the standard—note particularly the positioning of the much-used cursor and ENTER keys. A configuration that is ideal for one user or application may not be as comfortable or convenient for others. Also, needs vary if you use a mouse or other input device.

Another way to reduce keyboarding is to use voice commands to execute sequences or keystrokes or mouse actions. Voice recognition technology has improved greatly in recent years, as indicated by the low-cost but efficient Voice Master expansion card and headset from Covox shown in Figure 3. You can also use the computer's printer port to hook up this capacity for one spoken word to replace literally hundreds of keystrokes.

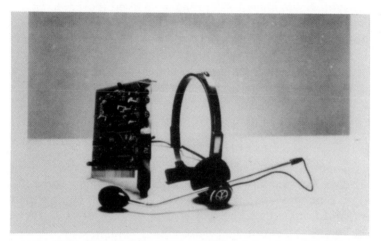

**Figure** **3.** Voice Master expansion card and headset from Covox.

A lot more attention is now given to keyboard ergonomics, and some new designs are proving effective at reducing typing stress.

If you are new to typing, then you can avoid the extra finger movements and inefficiency imposed by the traditional keyboard with the QWERTY configuration of keys, which was designed originally to slow down fast typists who could overtake and jam the mechanism of the early mechanical typewriters. Ergonomically more satisfactory is a DVORAK configuration, in which the most-used keys are placed where they are easiest to reach. You can buy DVORAK keyboards or use software to reconfigure the layout of the keys on a conventional keyboard.

The easiest way to reduce keyboarding is to make efficient use of mouse commands. Many software programs now take advantage of mouse control. You can also add mouse power to most word processing, spreadsheet, and other keyboarding-intensive programs by such devices as the PowerMouse (Figure 4) from ProHance Technologies. It puts many keyboard functions onto keys incorporated in an enlarged mouse. You can create macros that convert many keystrokes into far fewer hand and finger movements using the mouse.

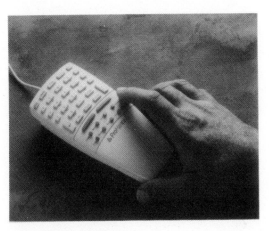

**Figure** 4. The ProHance mouse.

The problem with intensive and prolonged mouse operation is that your fingers and hands must continually make fine, precise movements. There is a tendency to cramp up the hand and wrist, creating the internal stress and lack of natural function that can bring on RSI problems similar to those caused by keyboarding.

In theory, trackballs are ergonomically better than mice. They are, in effect, mice turned upside down. That means you roll the ball with the fingertips or the palm of your hand instead of having to grasp the mouse and move it across the work surface. The control buttons that are on the top of the mouse are positioned in various ways on the top or sides of the trackball casing.

You may find a good trackball well suited to your computer work needs and habits, but many who have tried them have found them more tiring and awkward than the conventional mouse.

Other inputting devices include a whole new generation of touch pads and touch screens. It pays to experiment and keep up with the technology. However, no hardware is as beneficial as adopting correct posture and work habits if you do not want to become another RSI victim.

# 5

# *Exercise: The Solution to Most Computer Health Problems*

The most effective and easiest way to prevent most computer-related health problems is to exercise regularly. Exercise is *the* big health protection payoff, both for computer operators and the organizations that employ them.

Introducing short work breaks at least every two hours and training operators how to exercise properly during these breaks, as well as periodically while working, will reduce medical expenses and lost working time, while increasing productivity.

Computer-operating employees who exercise are a good business investment. Human resources are usually the single most important asset to any business. Preventive health strategies for people are more important than preventive maintenance for machines. Every successful company lubricates, cleans, and maintains its essential machines. Comparatively few look after their people as well.

On the following pages are special exercises for people who operate computers for long periods. Use them yourself to protect your own health, or use them as the basis for a preventive health strategy for your computer operators.

The exercises are designed both to prevent problems from arising and to aid your recovery if you have sustained damage.

## Exercise Anywhere

You may do these exercises while at work or at home, or you can add them to a general fitness regime. You can perform some of our exercises at the desk, others during short work breaks, others when walking, waiting for a bus or train, or other convenient times. The postural exercises can be done any time when you are sitting. If used regularly, these exercises will help to reduce stress and increase your overall productivity. So do not think of the time spent doing them as "lost" work time. They can actually contribute to increasing your work output substantially.

In other words, these exercises are cost-effective. If you are the computer operator, or you are reading this book because you manage date processing activities, accept exercising regularly at work as an investment in increasing both the quality and quantity of work output. These exercises can be a better investment in many computing situations than investing hundreds—even thousands—of dollars on upgrading your hardware or software.

These are low-stress exercises, to be undertaken gently in a relaxed way. They will not make you puff for breath, or increase your heart rate substantially. Nor will they cause you to perspire heavily—which is an important advantage when you need to exercise while wearing normal working clothes.

Consequently, these exercises should be suitable for any age. Many of them can be undertaken by computer users with physical handicaps. Of course, if you have any medical problem, are advanced in years, or there is some other reason why exercise of any kind might have negative consequences for you, then consult your doctor before you begin.

For virtually all of us, appropriate exercise is beneficial. It reduces stress and computer injuries and is believed to activate the endorphins, the body's natural, safe way to combat overload. Remarkable results in easing headaches and a whole range of other health problems are reported by computer users who exercise regularly. Get into the habit of doing these simple stretching and joint-easing routines whenever you have an opportunity. They really do help to make you feel—and work—better.

---

℞

# Quick Fix #18

Walking for half an hour each day can dramatically improve your health. For many workers, one of the easiest ways to do this is to incorporate walking into a commuting routine. Get off the subway or bus one stop early, walk to and from the station, park the car farther away from work, and so on. Try to take these walks without carrying heavy purses, briefcases, or other items that might involve your hands, wrists, or arms. Change your schedule so that there is adequate time for walking—you will lose many of the benefits of this gentle, natural exercise if you are pressured to meet a time deadline. Make walking time *quality* time for both your mind and body. Use it also to relax and exercise your computing-stressed eyes. Let them roam to take in the details of everything around you.

If extending your commute is not practical, or you work from home, then you should allocate thirty minutes every day to recreational walking. If you have a dog to accompany you, that can become a routine you will be reminded of every day!

---

## Getting Started

We suggest that you read through the descriptions of all the exercises first. Then try those that seem the most appropriate for you. Use them for a week, then read over the exercises again and experiment with some of the others. It will be helpful to you to be familiar with all the exercises because they have different purposes. You need to select from them a repertoire that will meet your particular needs at different times.

Before you begin, understand that it is quite usual when doing stretching exercises for one side of the body to feel tighter than the other, particularly if you sit awkwardly at your computer station and angle your body to one side. You will benefit from maintaining the stretch position on the tighter side for slightly longer during the exercises. Soon, as your joints become more flexible and your muscles both more stretched and relaxed, such localized conditions will become less noticeable.

Some of the exercises can be done in a sitting position. To get the best results, it is necessary that you sit upright and not slouch or incline your body or head forward or backward. If exercises do not stipulate that they should be done sitting or lying down, they should be performed in a standing position.

If you concentrate first on the exercises marked with an asterisk, you will follow an easy planned routine to better health. Later you can modify your routine, perhaps adding other exercises according to your individual needs. The purpose of the exercises with asterisks is similar to that of a software program's quick start instructions. Together, they get you up and running immediately and will demonstrate the program's benefits.

## Wrists and Hands

This group of exercises can be done sitting or standing. Remember that wrists and hands should not function in isolation from the arms or upper body. That applies when exercising as well as when working. Improving the health of your neck and shoulders will also help your hands and wrists to stay healthy despite the thousands of keyboard strokes or mouse movements you make during a typical working day.

The muscles in your arms are the main movers of your fingers and wrists, so while many of theses exercises seem focused on the arms, they are of direct benefit to your fingers, wrists, and hands.

*1. *Arm Stretches.* Position your right arm palm down and straight out in front of you parallel to the floor. With your left hand, gently pull the fingers of the right hand back toward your head. This will stretch those hand and arm muscles that become overused with lots of keyboarding. Do this at least twice daily, stretching both arms each time. Use this exercise also after you have been working at the keyboard for a long time or using a mouse intensively, e.g., doing CAD or desktop-publishing layout work.

*2. *Arm Massage.* Massage, gently but deeply, the muscles of your forearms. (See discussion later in this chapter for a description of how to massage yourself most effectively.) This may seem a very simple exercise and almost too easy to do, yet you will find it extremely effective in reducing cumulative stress in your arms and hands. Try to do it at least twice daily, more often if possible.

*3. *Hand Massage.* Massage the small muscles of your hand and fingers for a few minutes at least twice daily.

4. *Wrist Resistors.* With fingers out in front of you and palms facing down, gently push your hand backward against the pressure of mild resistance from the other hand. Allow your wrist to return to the neutral position without resistance. Repeat four times, with both hands. (When you type, you use predominantly the muscles on the underside of your arm, so they become inordinately strong. This exercise will strengthen the opposing muscles and balance and strengthen your wrist and hand function.)

(A similar exercise using a weight to strengthen these muscles is suggested by many doctors and therapists. Using a weight in this way is *not* appropriate for computer users. Holding the weight contracts muscles that are already very tight from keyboarding and resists the necessary strengthening of the *opposing* muscle groups.)

5. *Hand Shake.* Keeping your shoulders relaxed, gently shake out your hands. Imagine you have just washed them, there is no towel, and you are shaking off drops of water. Your hands can be in front of you or hanging down at your sides. Do this exercise whenever you can, for example when you pause from keyboarding to read from the screen.

6. *Hand Stretch.* With arms straight out in front of you, alternate closing and opening your hands as you move your straight arms up and down in a scissor pattern. The important aspect of this exercise is to stretch your hands and fingers as far as you can. Try to do this at least once a day.

7. *Thumb Stretch.* Move your thumb gently in toward your little finger and then stretch it out as far toward the back of your hand as you can. Do this four times for each thumb at least four times a day.

8. *Wrist Stretch.* With the thumb and fingers of one hand, grasp the other hand and gently exert traction on the wrist (that is, pull in a controlled, gentle, steady way). Imagine that the hand you are grasp-

ing is divided down the middle into two parts, so that you grasp and pull each part in turn. This will gently stretch each side of the wrist. Do this exercise four times daily.

9. *Finger Circles.* Begin with your arms relaxed at your sides. Then bend your arms at right angles, with your palms down. Holding your fingers straight but relaxed, make finger circles with one finger at a time. Do this several times in a clockwise direction, and then several times counterclockwise. Keep the other fingers still as best you can and move only the finger you are working on. Do this to all the fingers of both hands twice daily.

## Neck

Try the following exercises for the neck.

*1. *Straighten Up No. 1.* Standing with your back to a wall, straighten up by pressing the back of your head toward and into the wall. Move your head backward in a straight line, taking care not to bend your neck backward or raise your chin to enable your head to touch the wall. Be sure to tuck your chin in slightly and stretch the back of your neck upward as you do this exercise.

You may find that, without lifting your chin, the slouch in your shoulders and the forward positioning of your head that can result from prolonged desk or computer work make it difficult—even impossible—to get your head back beyond your shoulders to make contact with the wall. In that case, just move your head back as far as it will go without lifting your chin. Persist with this exercise three times daily and you should find that it becomes easier and your natural upright posture is gradually restored.

*2. *Straighten Up No. 2.* When sitting, standing, or walking, stretch your head and neck upward—as if you are trying to lengthen the back of your neck. Keep your chin slightly tucked in and reach up with the top of your head, as if there is a string gently pulling from the crown of your head. Repeat this exercise whenever you can. Make it a habit and your posture will improve rapidly.

3. *Neck Flexors.* Lie down comfortably on your back. Raise your head up by tucking in your chin and then curling your head up and

around toward your chest and then moving back to the original resting position. If there is any pain, then you are probably lifting your head up too far. In that case, try making smaller movements, gradually increasing them as the neck muscles become stronger. Do this exercise four to eight times, both morning and evening.

*4. *The Towel Roll.* This relaxation and stretching exercise is amazingly effective in relieving stiffness and other discomfort in the neck, shoulders, and upper back after long periods at the computer. It may seem like a simple back stretch, but it is fundamental in correcting the forward-bending posture that causes so many neck, arm, and hand problems among computer users.

Lie on your back—preferably on a carpeted floor—with a tightly rolled-up towel placed across your back and about three inches below your shoulder blades. Start with about a three-inch-diameter roll, increasing the thickness as you get used to the exercise.

Rest in this position for fifteen minutes, preferably twice daily. It is best if you don't read or talk on the phone while doing this exercise. Relax and focus on your breathing, allowing your chest to fall as you exhale. You may find this relaxing exercise fits in with your routine most easily if you do it first thing in the morning after waking up and last thing at night before going to bed.

A variation is to move the roll slightly higher so that it is at the base of your neck. Then your head will fall back naturally of its own weight until it reaches the bed, mat, floor, or whatever surface you are lying on. This applies gentle traction to the neck, helping to release overstressed neck muscles.

You can allocate a towel specifically for this exercise, keeping it rolled up with strong rubber bands. Or you may want to create a permanent neck roll. One way is to wrap duct tape tightly around a piece of plastic foam to form a cylinder of the appropriate size and stiffness. Cover the cylinder in an attractively colored or patterned cloth slipcase that can be removed for washing. This makes a great neck support for travel also.

5. *Shoulder Extensions.* Standing with your back to the wall and your arms in an L shape out at your sides, slide your arms up until they are stretched straight up over your head. Then bring them back to the starting position and repeat four times. You will feel the benefit of this exercise mostly in your shoulders and upper back. It is very helpful in developing the strength and flexibility in your shoulders

necessary for holding your head in a healthy position when computing. Do this four times daily.

(*The following neck exercises can be carried out sitting or standing.*)

6. *The Puppet String.* Imagine that there is a string at the top of your head gently pulling you upward. This will help you to sit up straight and so reduce the strain on your back and neck. Do this exercise as often as you can, especially while working at the computer.

*7. *Neck Extensions.* Clasp your fingers behind your head, with the elbows pointed forward. Gently extend your head backward against the natural resistance created by your hands. Offer no resistance when bringing your head back to the starting position. Repeat this exercise five times on about three occasions each day.

8. *Neck Massage No. 1.* Massage the small muscles at the bottom inch of the back of your skull. Do this for a minute or two twice a day to reduce head and neck tension.

9. *Neck Massage No. 2.* Massage the small muscles at the top of your neck, where they meet the skull, twice daily.

10. *Neck Massage No. 3.* Massage with moderate force the muscles on the back and sides of your neck twice daily.

11. *Neck Stretches.* Imagine there is a clock face on the floor and you are sitting in the center of it, facing the twelve o'clock position. Breathe in a relaxed way. Allow your head to fall forward gently toward the twelve o'clock position. Feel the stretching that results from allowing your neck to relax and be gently pulled by the weight of your head.

With your head still hanging forward, move it slowly in a circular motion so that you pause for a few seconds at the one-thirty, three o'clock, four-thirty, six o'clock, seven-thirty, nine o'clock, ten-thirty, and twelve o'clock positions. As you rest on each of these positions feel the stretch created by the weight of your head.

Pause for a few moments with your head up in the resting position, balanced vertically over your shoulders and facing twelve o'clock. Then drop your head forward again repeating the exercise in the opposite direction. Be sure to go slowly and gently.

If you encounter an uncomfortable or sore position, stay there for slightly longer so that the stretching action can help to adjust distortion in your neck muscles and joints. Repeat twice daily.

*12. *Relaxing and Balancing Your Head and Neck.* Just relax and concentrate on the sensation created by the weight of your head resting on the top of your neck, together with the weight of your head and neck resting on your shoulders. Now become conscious of the weight of your head and how to find the best position to hold it so that it is balanced without any effort on your neck and shoulders.

Imagine the point where the head balances on the neck to be a ball on the tip of a triangle. Make this another good posture habit, so that you habitually adopt this position unconsciously all the time.

## Shoulders

These shoulder exercises are very beneficial to your neck also.

1. *The Crane.* Imagine you are a stately, slender bird spreading your wings. Stand with your arms hanging loosely at your sides. Bring them up so that they cross in front of your chest, then gently swing them out to the sides, with one rising high and one low. Do this several times, alternating the arm held high and the one held low. Repeat two or three times a day.

*(The next seven exercises can be done sitting or standing.)*

2. *Shoulder Stretches No. 1.* Raise the palm of one hand so that it is facing and about 6–8 inches in front of your forehead. With the other hand, pull your elbow across your body toward the opposite shoulder. Feel the shoulder, and particularly the shoulder blades, stretch away from your torso. Repeat with each side four times twice a day.

*3. *Arm Circles.* With a relaxed straight arm, trace a large circle in the air with your fingertips so that your shoulder rotates in as full a circle as possible. Do this in both directions with one arm several times, and then repeat several times with the other arm. Repeat twice daily.

*4. *Tightening the Wings No. 1.* Tighten your upper back so that your shoulder blades move close together; hold this position for a moment, then release it. Repeat four times twice daily.

5. *Shoulder Circles.* Slowly rotate both shoulders forward in a full circle four times and then back in the opposite direction four times. Then rotate each shoulder separately. Do this twice daily.

6. *Shoulder Releasing.* Inhale gently as you draw your shoulders up toward your ears. Exhale completely, allowing your shoulders to drop with the weight of your arms. Repeat this exercise at intervals throughout the day.

7. *Releasing Stress.* With arms hanging at your sides and your fingers gently pointing toward the floor, inhale deeply and visualize that you are gathering up all your tensions. When you exhale, imagine all this tension running out of your fingertips into the ground. If you are doing this correctly, you should feel the weight of your arms pulling downward as you exhale. Repeat this routine three times at intervals throughout the day, especially when you need to relieve stress and mental or emotional tension.

*8. *Reaching Up.* Stand with both arms reaching straight above your head. Now reach with one hand as high as you can and feel the stretching in your shoulder muscles and under your arm. Repeat the same motion with the other arm, alternating sides about five times each. Do this twice a day.

9. *Tightening the Wings No. 2.* Stand with your back against a wall. Push your shoulders back into the wall. Hold this position for a moment and then release. Repeat six times twice daily.

*10. *Loosening the Wings.* Place the underside edge of your forearm flat against a door frame and lean your upper body a short distance into the doorway. You should feel a stretch in your shoulder and under your arm. Repeat with the other arm. Do this exercise twice every day (or more frequently, for example every time you go through the door of your office or the bathroom).

11. *Shoulder Stretches.* Lie on your back on the floor with your knees up, your feet on the ground, and your arms crossed over your stomach. Keeping your lower back flat on the floor, reach out sideways with your arms so that they rest on the floor with the palms up, stretching straight out to the sides. Rest a few moments to allow the stretching to take effect. Now cross your arms again and reach them out about twelve inches higher, then twelve inches higher again, and then straight above your head. In some of these positions your shoulders may feel very tight and your arms may not be able to rest on the floor. This is all right, as your shoulders will stretch by doing this exercise once or twice a day, and so it will become progressively easier.

12. *Finger-Walking.* Stand facing a wall, about two feet in front of it. Walk the fingertips of one hand up the wall as high as you can go. Return to the neutral position. Now turn at right angles and repeat, standing sideways to the wall and about two feet away from it. This is an excellent exercise if you have shoulder pain or your shoulders are very tight. Do it twice every day.

Mark the top point that your fingers reach and try to walk your fingers 1 inch higher up the wall every week. This provides a visual record of your improvement and gives you incentive to stretch farther.

## Releasing Lower-Back Tension

The following exercises are designed to release lower-back tension.

*1. *Pelvic Tilts.* Lie on your back with your knees bent and feet on the floor. Tighten your belly so that your pelvis tilts up, then releases. Do this ten to fifteen times twice every day.

*2. *Fetal Position.* While lying on your back, lace your fingers around your knees and gently pull them toward your chest. Do not cross your ankles. Inhale slowly and deeply into your lower back, feeling it lengthen as you exhale. Do this once or twice every day.

3. *Lower-Abdominal Sit-Ups.* Start with the same position as the Pelvic Tilts exercise. With your knees apart and your toes pointed slightly inward, curl up your pelvis and hold it there throughout this exercise. With your hands clasped behind your head, do quarter sit-ups. (These are less strenuous than full sit-ups because you do not have the strain of coming up to a full sitting position.) Do five to twenty at a time, depending on your strength level. Then rest for twenty seconds. Do three sets, twice daily.

This exercise is very important to establish lower-back strength and stability and will help to relieve the pressure on your neck from long-term computing.

*4. *Hamstring Stretches.* (*Select and incorporate twice a day into your exercise routine* at least one *of the four exercises that follow. Consult your health practitioner if you experience any burning pain in your leg when doing a hamstring stretch.*)

- Sit on the edge of your chair after you have pushed it back from your desk. Extend one of your straightened legs out in front of you, with your toes pointing toward the ceiling. Bend forward from your waist, keeping your back straight. You should feel a pull behind your extended leg, sometimes also in your hip and lower back. Hold for four to five relaxed breaths and repeat with the other leg. Do this four times daily.
- Sit on the floor with both legs out in front of you. Keeping your back as straight as possible, reach forward with your hands and grab your toes. If you cannot reach your toes, hold a towel between your hands and hook it over the balls of your feet. Hold for four or five relaxed breaths. Do this twice daily.
- Sit on the floor with one leg straight, toes pointing toward the ceiling. Bend your other leg at the knee, with your foot in front of where you are sitting. With your back straight, reach over and grab the foot of the extended leg. Use a towel if you need to extend your reach. Do both legs. Repeat twice daily.
- Standing, put the heel of one straightened leg on a stair, stool, chair, or desk top, depending on your degree of flexibility. Your toe must be pointing toward the ceiling, and the foot you are standing on must be pointing in the same direction as the extended leg. Bend slightly forward at the waist, keeping your back straight, and hold the stretch for four to five breaths. Do both legs twice a day.

5. *Calf Stretch.* Stand on the ball of one foot near the edge of a stair. Allow the heel to drop below the edge of the stair so that it is below the level of your toe and stretching the calf muscle. (You should probably hold on to something to maintain your balance.) Now push up with your foot so that you are again standing with all your weight on the ball of the foot. Then drop into the stretch again. Stretch both legs this way once a day.

6. *Sitting Up.* While sitting up with both feet flat on the floor, push your feet firmly into the ground. Feel how this causes your back to lift up. It is very helpful in correcting the slouched position created by computer work. Be sure to keep your buttocks relaxed as you do this. Repeat throughout the day.

7. *Flattening the Back.* Lie on your back with knees bent and your feet on the floor. With your arms stretched straight over the top of your head and your palms up, press the small of your back into the floor.

Hold for a count of one breath and relax. Do this several times. This also stretches your shoulders and upper back.

8. *Resting the Lower Back.* Lie on the floor with your legs on the seat of a chair. Slide your buttocks slightly under the chair so that your knees are pointing a little toward your head. Inhale, drawing your breath deeply into your lower back. Relax as you exhale.

9. *Twists.* Lie on your back with your legs out in front of you. Slide one leg up at the side, keeping it on the floor, until the knee is approximately at a right angle to your body. Raise the knee, bringing it over and across the middle of your body, then hold it with the opposite hand. Reach the hand on the same side as the bent knee straight out to the side, and turn your head to this side also. Hold for three to four breaths and then repeat with the other side.

10. *Roll Downs.* Standing with your feet about shoulder width apart, drop your head forward and let your body bend over forward so that you are rolling down the spine, one vertebra at a time. Your arms should hang relaxed at your sides. Bend your knees slightly as you straighten up by rolling back up, one vertebra at a time. Repeat three times twice a day.

11. *Leg Pulls.* Standing on one leg, bend the other behind you. Grab the foot of the bent leg with the opposite hand, and gently pull it toward your back. (You should hold on to a doorknob or desk for support.) This will stretch the front of the thigh and is important for the health of the lower back of the computer user.

12. *Partial Knee Bends.* During work breaks, stand with arms hanging relaxed at your sides and bend your knees. While keeping the buttocks relaxed and your body upright, push your feet into the floor to bring your body into an upright standing position. Repeat four to eight times.

This exercise helps to strengthen the lower back. If it is difficult for you to go down very far, you will find it easier if you stand with your heels on a block of wood or a book about 1.5–2 inches high.

## Doorknob Exercises

Every home or office has lots of exercise aids. You do not need to buy expensive equipment, and you can find opportunities to exercise almost anywhere, anytime. Among the most effective of these readily available exercise accessories is the humble doorknob. Here are two special doorknob exercises.

1. With your hand positioned as if you were going to shake hands with someone, grab a doorknob. Lean away from it sideways, allowing the shoulder and shoulder blade to pull and stretch away from the body. You may need to rotate your body a little, forward or backward, to get the best stretch. Repeat three to four times a day. (This is one of our favorites.)

2. Position yourself the same as for the first exercise, but this time rotate your chest outward so that the space between your shoulder and chest widens. This is a good stretching exercise for the upper chest and shoulder. Repeat it twice daily.

## A Good Night's Sleep

Your body does not go into suspended animation when you sleep; you carry the stresses and physical tension of the day into your sleeping hours. So extend the good things you seek to achieve from your exercise routine and healthy work habits into your sleeping hours.

Exercise will stretch out your tight muscles and relax your breathing before you retire for the night. Taking a walk also contributes to a good night's sleep.

Don't sleep on your stomach; it will strain your neck and can aggravate a sore lower back. If your lower back is painful or tired, sleep on your back with two or three pillows under your knees to elevate them.

If you are more comfortable sleeping on your side, put a 2- to 3-inch pillow between your knees to keep them separated through the night. Doing this may help relieve pain in your lower back. You may also want to put a small rolled-up towel underneath your waist to give it additional support throughout the night, if you are in pain.

## Massage

Massage is an effective treatment for chronic muscle strain, stress, and even fatigue. Treatment from a qualified massage therapist can help tune up a stressed professional, but what we are addressing here is self-massage for your hands, arms, neck, shoulders, and around the eyes as a form of preventive and remedial therapy.

If the muscles you are massaging are small, use the pads of your fingers and thumb to work specific areas. When dealing with large muscles, use your whole hand to knead the tight muscles with gentle, fluid strokes.

If massaging is painful at first, reduce both the force and the period of treatment, massaging gently for more frequent but shorter periods. Increase the force and duration of the massage as it becomes more comfortable to do so.

Sometimes when muscles have been locked in spasm—stuck in contraction—for long periods of time they will feel sore when they begin to soften and become more healthy. This pain is temporary and natural. It happens because chemical irritants are locked into the muscle tissues owing to the severe inhibition of blood circulation in spasmed muscles. Circulation is restored as the muscle contraction softens, and these irritants begin to circulate into the surrounding tissues as they are flushed away.

Massage (and exercise) will release these irritants, sometimes causing pain and soreness until they are flushed away by healthy circulation. If this occurs, you can help your body through this period more quickly by drinking additional amounts of water (distilled if possible) throughout the day. This increases the intercellular fluid level and helps to wash away the congested particles.

# 6

# *Eat Well to Compute Better*

Diet and nutrition are vital to your computing health. Spending much of your time in sedentary, highly intense computing activities creates specific nutritional needs while, at the same time, exposing you to the temptation of many bad dietary habits.

This chapter examines some of the basic dietary pitfalls that are probably affecting your career—and other facets of your life—in strongly negative ways. You are probably not aware of these dangers, but they are as real as other computing-related health problems. In fact, they may be far more dangerous to you than the invisible electromagnetic radiation emanating from your VDT.

There is much you can do at very little inconvenience or cost to remedy dietary hazards. The payoff is immediate. Better eating results directly in a higher quality of both working and leisure life.

What follows is not yet another lecture on eating healthy foods— you have probably heard enough preaching on that subject already! We treat you as we would an athlete seeking practical aids to better performance. As a computer user, you have particular nutritional needs because of the work you do. These needs are not necessarily the same as those of other workers, any more than the nutritional requirements for a sprinter are the same as those for one who lifts weights.

So in this chapter we suggest what you should eat and drink to enable you to think better and work more productively at the keyboard. Even more important, if you follow these suggestions, they will help to minimize your exposure to many of the health risks inherent in computer work.

You also may avoid adding unnecessary weight, and even lose surplus fat that has already accumulated from unhealthy eating habits at the keyboard.

## GIGO: Garbage In, Garbage Out

Many of us become so preoccupied with the work we are doing on our computers that we give little thought to the food we put into our bodies. The temptation is enormous to snack on convenience and junk food, drink a lot of coffee and sodas, and ingest large amounts of sugar. We have neither the time nor the inclination to think much about what we eat when we are working or playing with our fascinating machines.

A standard measure of the quality of computer hardware is the amount of downtime during which it is inoperative because of some fault or other. Downtime is expensive and can create all kinds of adverse consequences. You minimize hardware downtime by protecting your hardware from physical abuse, particularly from additional stress caused by "dirty" electrical power, in which the voltage and current may vary considerably from the ideal for which the hardware is designed.

Similarly, you minimize your body's "downtime"—the periods during which it will not function properly—by ensuring that its power input is as near as possible to the ideal for which it was designed. That power input is in the form of the food you eat and the air you breathe. They comprise the body's fuel, which is needed as much for efficient thinking as for the physical actions of hitting keys. So it needs to be as clean and pure as possible.

## Air: The Number One Fuel

The air that we breathe is our number one fuel, essential for the proper functioning of the brain and all the other components of the body. We can go for many days without eating, and quite a long time without drinking, but if our breathing is restricted, most of us will die within three minutes.

So we urge you to give due regard to the information in this book dealing with exercise and breathing. A diet strategy that is not combined with attention to breathing and exercise cannot be fully effective.

---

℞

## Quick Fix #19

Whenever you eat or drink, inhale and exhale gently and deeply five times, both before and after. Try not to eat and drink while actually working. Instead, use the opportunity to take a break, stretch your body, and relax and deepen your breathing.

Try not to ingest excess air with food or drink, as this can cause flatulence and discomfort. Chew the food well with your mouth closed, and swallow fluids slowly so that you do not take too much air into your stomach. Some people with digestive problems find it helpful to drink after, rather than during, a meal.

---

### Food and Drink

Our second most important energy input comes from the food and drink we consume. They can reduce our performance and cause damage if they are of the wrong type, in the incorrect quantities, or consumed at unsuitable intervals.

Like your computer, your body needs power surge protection. Sharp fluctuations in the electrical power supply to your computer can garble data, even damage or destroy sensitive electronic components. Food and drink form the energy supply to your body, and the body needs to be protected from unregulated energy surges resulting from the food and drink you consume. These surges, like the microtrauma we discussed in Chapter 4, have a cumulative effect that can damage, even destroy, your body components.

The main causes of energy surges in the body are caffeine—as found in coffee, tea, and many soft drinks—and sugar. The habitual use of coffee and sugar weaken the body, lower your energy level, and reduce your productivity. You greatly increase your health risks and lower the quality of the work you do if consuming large quantities of caffeine and sugar is one of your computing habits.

Consider for a moment what the coffee in the cup alongside your keyboard, or that Danish or candy bar, does to your energy level when you work at your computer.

The adrenal glands are the regulators of body energy, making it available in a controlled way to maintain a balanced energy level over time, rather than in peaks and valleys that make you swing between the extremes of feeling energetic and exhausted. The habitual use of caffeine and sugar plays havoc with the natural balancing mechanism of the adrenal glands. You get a demonstration of this when you experience the increased alertness and surge of energy that follows drinking a cup of coffee or eating a candy bar. If you drink coffee and eat sweet things throughout the day, you artificially stimulate the adrenal glands to keep on triggering releases of energy into the body. This is in the form of glycogen released into the bloodstream. The result is a high that is similar in many respects to the boost from various addictive drugs.

As with illicit drugs, after a time the highs are not really highs at all. Your body is operating in such an unnatural, inefficient, subnormal way that the energy kicks you get from the caffeine and sugar do not even bring you up to the level of performance and the feeling of well-being that should be your normal state.

Substances such as coffee, sugar, and certain drugs that appear to give you energy actually *steal* it. They trigger the body to dig deeper into its own energy reserves and release the stored energy that nature has wisely designed for us to conserve for real emergencies, such as life-threatening crises or a work situation that demands quick thought and action.

By drinking coffee and sweetened soft drinks and eating candy bars throughout the day, you create a run on your energy bank deposits. There is a succession of highs and lows that do not give your body a chance to catch up with itself and maintain a natural, balanced state. You soon go beyond your body's energy credit limit and become continually stressed.

The food and drink you consume sends your body false emergency signals similar to those it receives naturally from external stimuli, such as a work crisis or some threat in your environment. Consequently, your body chemistry goes haywire and your body malfunctions, as would an engine misfiring because it is running on bad fuel or is overloaded by unregulated electrical power.

So the stresses inherent in computer work are aggravated by bad habits that include the frequent ingestion of stimulants such as caffeine and sugars. The damage caused by bad diet builds, accumulating into a number of potentially serious health conditions. These stimulants cause your body and your mind to operate inefficiently.

## Quick Fix #20

As a computer user, you have an easy way to monitor what you are actually getting when you eat convenience foods from such leading national outlets as McDonald's, Dairy Queen, Domino's, and Wendy's.

You can use software programs to learn the ingredients and help you manage your dietary intake.

For example, FASTFOOD by Pat Archey and Bud Branchflower gives a quick ready reference to scores of taste temptations available all over the United States. You can also get programs on diet from bulletin boards and shareware libraries. FASTFOOD and the companion program, Nutrition Manager, which enables you to analyze your entire diet, are also available direct from PBCShare Inc., P.O. Box 70531, Bellevue, Washington 98007 (206/641-7390). (If you find the programs useful, a modest registration fee of about $20 is requested by the authors.)

## Sugar: Public Enemy Number One

As someone who uses a computer extensively, you operate your body in ways that make it particularly vulnerable to excess sugar. Indeed, sugar is the computer operator's number one enemy and makes us susceptible to obesity, stress-related problems, diabetes, and other undesirable health conditions.

Biologically, sugar is the trigger for the appetite mechanism in the human body. When your blood sugar drops below a certain point, you feel hungry. In the old days, before processed junk food was available, this natural mechanism worked fine. Throughout most of human history, the food available to us has contained only small amounts of natural sugar, so until processed foods became so readily available, it was almost impossible to overindulge in sugar. Our natural occasional craving for something sweet was just nature's way to help us achieve a balanced diet.

When we sought sugar satisfaction from natural foods, we predominantly ingested starch, a form of carbohydrate. Starch is made up of long and complex molecules that break down and reach the bloodstream slowly, over an extended period. It is the equivalent of a slow-burning fuel. So starch provides a sustained and even energy level from your food, unlike processed sugar, which shoots your energy level up for a short time, after which it quickly drops down again.

Nutritionists emphasize that our bodies are not designed to handle the large intakes of sugar that result in these energy surges. But in modern life temptation is everywhere. In these days of readily available processed food and intense pressure on our time, when we feel hungry we go for fast foods, which often contain large amounts of processed sugar. Sugar in a concentrated and very potent form is absorbed quickly, causing our blood sugar level to rise rapidly. This may give an immediate short burst of energy, even a temporary feeling of euphoria, but this effect is followed by a let-down in the form of tiredness, and a feeling of weakness, sometimes even mental depression.

This chain reaction traps us in "the sugar cycle." The feelings of weakness, tiredness, and mental depression will trigger the desire for another fix of sugar. So the regular excess intake of sugar in our diet becomes a form of addiction.

The remedy is to eat instead the complex carbohydrates found in whole grains, vegetables, and whole fruits. They supply an even, stable form of energy for your body and mind to work most efficiently. This will give you greater staying power when working at the keyboard— and in all other aspects of your life.

Another adverse consequence of the sugar cycle is that we reduce our natural feelings of hunger, yet gain almost no nourishment from the candies, pastries, and many other sugar-rich products that we consume. The symptoms of the hunger urge are satisfied by eating sugar, but the body's need for nourishment is not met. Processed sugar contains no minerals, protein, or vitamins. It is an empty food, and when we eat it we incur a nutritional debt. Indeed, not only does excess sugar not contribute to our energy resources, it actually depletes them further.

Sugar cannot be metabolized—broken down into usable constituents— in your body unless the necessary vitamins, minerals, protein, and fat are present. When you develop an excess sugar consumption pattern, these metabolism-supporting nutrients are not provided as they would be in a balanced diet, so they must be taken from the reserves within your body. This leaves your body increasingly deficient in these vital substances.

Consequently, a high proportion of Americans—especially those of us in sedentary occupations such as computing—are overfed yet nutritionally deficient at the same time. As computer users, we are particularly vulnerable to the sugar cycle, and so should study food packaging carefully to keep our total sugar consumption down as much as possible. (Empty sugars are disguised under a variety of names on food labels, including sucrose, fructose, glucose, maltose, dextrose, lactose, and corn syrup.) You can do this in part by switching to artificial sweeteners, but they are not without hazards. Honey is a natural alternative and is absorbed relatively slowly, so it can be used in moderation as a sugar substitute. But you should drastically reduce all your sugar intake, including honey, to be healthier, both in body and mind.

## The Cholesterol Threat

There are good reasons to suspect that cholesterol levels are higher in computer users than in the general population because of our sedentary life-style and our dietary habits. Cholesterol comes mostly from fatty foods and is dangerous because excessive amounts in the diet can cause a buildup along the walls of the blood vessels and arteries. This decreases the size and flexibility of the vessels conveying blood throughout the body, aggravating the problems that many computer users already have from restricted blood circulation caused by bad posture and lack of exercise.

As cholesterol accumulates, the decreasing blood flow to organs and muscles reduces the body's efficiency, including the dispersal of irritants and waste products arising from stress and microtrauma. As we saw earlier, the accumulation of these irritants in joints and muscle tissue can be a cause of pain. So pain at the keyboard can be a symptom stemming directly from sustained bad eating habits.

The heart muscle itself may be damaged from blood circulation problems stemming directly from diet, leading to a heart attack. A piece of the plaque caused by cholesterol can break away from the wall of a blood vessel and obstruct one of the arteries that carry blood and major nutrients to the brain. This results in a stroke, which can permanently impair physical body functions, as well as the way that you think and communicate.

So there are many reasons to limit your fat intake significantly and try to keep your blood cholesterol levels as low as possible.

Many fast foods contain significant amounts of fat, particularly if they are fried. You should eliminate excessive amounts of saturated fats from your diet, for example by not eating fatty meats, whole milk, cream, butter, cheese, hydrogenated vegetable oil, and solid margarines.

Not all cholesterol is bad. Some is manufactured within the body to facilitate such essential tasks as the insulation of nerves, to help build defenses against infection, and as building blocks for sexual hormones. But extra cholesterol beyond the body's natural needs can be a great danger to your health.

## Beneficial Complex Carbohydrates

Complex carbohydrates are our major source of energy and should make up the bulk of our diet. By burning these carbohydrates through oxidation, we convert them to energy for the body. The diet suggestions at the end of this chapter are rich in complex carbohydrates that provide energy without the penalties that come from having too much sugar, fat, or cholesterol.

## Protein Pointers

Protein is the basic building block of all human tissue. It is the structure around which bone, muscle, and skin are developed, and it is essential in the repair mechanism of the body. But you can have too much of a good thing, and the typical American diet contains two to three times the daily dose of protein recommended for a healthy body.

A particularly damaging aspect of our protein-rich diets in developed countries is that we eat too much meat. As red meat often contains as much as 50 percent fat, it should be eliminated, or make up only a very minor part of your diet. Your protein needs can be met from other, healthier sources.

Another reason for cutting back on meat as a protein source is that modern methods of raising animals include feeding them hormone preparations so that they gain weight faster and are consequently more profitable. Farm animals are often given antibiotics as well. Residues of these drugs remain in the meat and so are taken into your own body.

Try to get most of your protein from tofu, chicken (without the skin, which is high in fat), fish, legumes (beans and peas), whole grains, and nuts.

## Food Additives and Your CPU

The critical component of your computer hardware that has most need for special protection from stress and damage is the central processing unit, which controls the whole system. Consequently, it is protected by fuses, surge suppressors, and ventilation. Similarly, we need to protect our own CPUs, our brains, which are very vulnerable to what we eat.

Of particular concern are the 2,000 or so chemicals used as food additives. Most of them have been tested to reduce the risk that they will do us serious physical harm, but we have very little evidence about their potential to upset the delicate chemical balances in our brains, which play such an important role in our memory and information processing functions.

In the 1950s, when the federal government eventually got around to legislating what additives could be put in foods to preserve, color, and flavor them, so many were already in common use that the cost of testing all of them was prohibitive. So a regulation was introduced that arbitrarily decided that those additives used before 1958 would be referred to as generally recognized as safe (GRAS), despite the fact that they had not been tested thoroughly. There are 768 of these GRAS additives, including preservatives, stabilizers, artificial flavors, and sweeteners. Their use is allowed without thorough testing.

As the use of processed and convenience fast foods skyrockets, we consume ever-increasing quantities of food additives. More than two to three pounds of these chemicals are swallowed by the typical American every year. There is a growing belief among pediatricians and psychiatrists that chemical additives and sugar contribute to behavior disorders. They seem to have particular effects on children, but they can also cause restlessness, difficulty in learning, and hyperactivity in adults.

So it is a wise precaution to take the time to read the list of contents of the processed foods you put into your precious body. Only an expert can be knowledgeable about even the most frequently used of the 2,000 food additives to which we are exposed, but we can all try to follow the maxim: If you don't know what it is, don't eat it!

## Water: The Liquid of Life

Water can be lethal to your computer electronics, but without it human beings cannot survive for more than a few days. Next to air, water is our most basic fuel. Yet very few computer users consume nearly enough water to sustain them during long, stressful work periods.

Water comprises about 70 percent of our body volume and is the main component of cells. Dehydrated cells cannot build healthy tissue or utilize energy efficiently. Toxins build up in the bloodstream because the fluid level is low, and circulation decreases, slowly poisoning you. Without adequate water intake, circulation is impaired, and oxygen and other necessary nutrients cannot be shipped efficiently to the areas of the body that need them. You become weakened, tired, and your mind loses its clarity.

Athletes who sweat profusely have clear signs that they should replenish their body fluid. It is just as important for a serious computer user to drink adequate water every day. You may not sweat as much running your spreadsheets or processing words as you would on the track, but you may need water just as much to maintain healthy, normal body functions.

The body is designed to run on water, not Classic Coke, tea, coffee, or beer. These commercial alternatives may be predominantly water, and taste great, but regular use of them may harm your health in several ways. For example, they may act as diuretics, causing your body to eliminate more fluid than you take in. Many of these commercial drinks also contain large quantities of processed sugar, along with flavorings and additives that may harm your health. Of course, the habitual use of alcohol and caffeine can become addictive.

Most adults do not have particularly sensitive thirst mechanisms, and so we may not be alerted sufficiently to our regular need for water. That is why it is important to drink water frequently as a habit, and not wait until you actually feel thirsty.

If the quality of your tap water is not great, buy bottled water or purchase a good quality water filter. Be sure to drink 6–8 glasses per day, more if you exercise regularly.

## Food for the Mind

Your psychological state affects how you eat, and how you eat affects your psychological state. If you eat well, you give your body and mind the best input to help you control your energy and your psychological and emotional ups and downs throughout the day. Many people are not aware of the connection between their feelings of restlessness, irritability, and tiredness and their habitual use of sugar, caffeine, and junk food.

The stomach and digestive problems of many computer users also are linked to the interaction between diet and mind. Such common ailments as ulcers, poor digestion, intestinal gas, diarrhea, and constipation relate directly to diet and may be aggravated further by a sedentary computing work style. Even healthy natural food will not be digested properly when you are highly stressed, upset or very tired, and sitting cramped in a bad posture for hours on end.

If the stomach or intestines are irritated from stress or poor diet, you will be prone to feeling more anxious. So another unhealthy cycle gathers momentum. But by becoming aware of the relationship between how you feel and the food you eat, you can take control of your diet in a way that will support your professional goals and overall health.

Follow a sensible diet and you will find that your general mental state, especially your clarity of thought, improves considerably. Diet particularly affects your stress level, which in turn is a major influence on all aspects of your physical and mental well being.

Eat for health and you can limit your stress considerably, even under intense pressures. By doing this you maintain a more even energy level, your body and emotions are stronger, and you will be less vulnerable to the external stresses that can affect our lives so profoundly.

## Reboot Your Body

You should be convinced by now that diet is very important for all computer users. To help you "reboot" and "reprogram" your body, try this twenty-point quick-start guide to healthier computing. It is a summary of useful information to help you get a quick start to a new and better life-style.

1. Eat less salt, refined sugar, and fat. Eat more fresh fruit, vegetables, whole grains, poultry, fish, and skim milk.

2. Eat lots of fresh or lightly steamed vegetables every day. They will nourish you well, supplying essential minerals and nutrients, and directly contribute to reducing stress. In addition, they are good for digestion, since roughage improves the tone of the intestinal muscles.

3. Exercise your jaws by chewing your food well to improve your digestion; your body will gain more nourishment from the food you eat.

4. Get regular! Many computer users seem to suffer from constipation, a consequence of posture, stress, lack of exercise, dehydration, and poor diet. The habitual use of laxatives creates a dependency on them, and bowel function becomes weakened. Fresh fruits and vegetables, and plenty of water, are nature's laxatives and also excellent sources of minerals, vitamins, and carbohydrates.

5. Limit your intake of breads, pastas, and pastries; they are empty nutritionally. When you satisfy your hunger by filling yourself with these foods, you deprive the body of the nutrition you would get from eating fresh, wholesome foods.

6. Substitute high-quality natural foods for processed convenience foods that have very little nutritional value and contain lots of sugar, food additives, and preservatives.

7. Use low-fat or skim milk and low-fat yogurt and cheese instead of their whole milk versions. This will help to reduce your overall fat intake. Try to eliminate dairy products as a main food source from your diet, using them only as adjuncts.

8. Cut down—or eliminate—red meats, replacing them with tofu, fresh fish, chicken (without the skin), whole grains, vegetables, and fruits. Tofu is an excellent source of protein, and it is easily digestible. Whole grains such as brown rice, barley, and millet give even-burning energy to the body, and so are very good for stabilizing the entire system.

9. Eat less, but often. The body uses calories more efficiently if they are taken in multiple small meals. A single large meal overloads the digestive system, and excess calories are stored as fat.

10. Avoid salt as it can lead to high blood pressure and fluid retention.

11. Break the habit of snacking at the keyboard, or at least ensure that eating while you work is less hazardous to your health. Instead of candy and potato chips, try raw unsalted nuts and sunflower seeds. (Be warned that if you eat a lot of nuts and do not drink adequate water, you may get constipated.)

12. Acquire a taste for bean sprouts and other natural convenience foods with high nutritional value. You can actually grow sprouts in a dish on your desk as a living snack on which to graze when computing!

13. Use yogurt and other naturally fermented milk products when digestion is troublesome. These foods can be helpful when you are under stress or recuperating from an illness. However, use them only a few times a week, rather than every day.

14. Remember that rye, pumpernickel, and whole wheat are among the most nutritious breads, but that any breads must be eaten only sparingly with your meals. They are filling and eating too much of them will satisfy your appetite, preventing you from eating the foods you need for nourishment.

15. When you get the sugar urge, eat fresh fruit, vegetables, nuts, or health food snack bars. (Many snack bars contain added sugar, so check the label to avoid this.)

16. Overall eat less quantity and more quality. Overeating can lead

to many health problems for computer users because of the sedentary work style.

17. Try to eat fiber-rich whole foods that increase your vitamin and mineral intake. This means more fruits, vegetables, whole grains, and beans. Generally, it is best for your computing health to choose foods like cereals, small orders of pastas, fruits, and lots of vegetables. They are your best fuel for the day.

18. Eat butter and ice cream in moderation, if at all. Besides being high in saturated fats, they are difficult to digest and can make you feel sluggish for hours after eating them.

19. Cut down—or eliminate—fried foods. They are difficult to digest, disturb your body chemistry and make you more irritable, and are a source of saturated fat, which may contribute to heart disease and stroke.

20. A good-quality natural multiple vitamin can be a great way to supply some of the nutrients missing in your diet.

## A Diet Menu Plan for Healthy Computing

Here is a diet menu plan for healthy eating to support intense hours at the computer. This is the outline of a basic, nonfanatical, healthy diet. Use it as you would a word processing style sheet or a database template to provide a structure, modifying it to your particular circumstances.

At each meal time, choose one food from each group—(a), (b), (c), (d), and (e). Lunch and dinner may be interchanged. In between meals you may want to snack on fresh fruits or raw nuts, small amounts of dried fruit, sugarless low-fat yogurt with fruit, or a sugarless health food snack bar.

*Breakfast*

(a) A glass of juice, preferably fresh (e.g., tomato, orange, grapefruit)
   or
   Fresh fruit (e.g., banana, orange, grapefruit, apple, grapes, papaya)
(b) Cereal (e.g., hot oatmeal, Wheatena, granola, shredded wheat)

with low-fat or skim milk and no sugar. You can add raisins for sweetness.
>    or
Small omelet
>    or
Two eggs (poached, boiled, or scrambled)
>    or
Low-fat cottage cheese
(c) One slice of toast
(d) Herb tea, decaffeinated beverage, or skim milk

*Lunch*

(a) Tomato juice, fresh fruit, or apple sauce
(b) Raw vegetable salad, including lettuce, spinach, cucumber, celery, carrot, tomato
>    or
Spinach salad
>    or
Soup and salad combination
>    or
Chicken or tuna salad
>    or
Tuna or chicken salad sandwich
>    or
Low-fat cottage cheese salad
>    or
Open-faced sandwich with lean meat (e.g., two thin slices of turkey)
(c) Small baked potato
>    or
Brown rice, kasha, bulgur, or barley
>    or
Cup of soup (not creamy soup, which is high in fat)
>    or
Small order of cole slaw
>    or
Small order of potato salad
>    or
Low-fat yogurt with fruit

(d) Lightly cooked vegetables
(e) Herb tea, decaffeinated beverage, or skim milk

*Dinner*

(a) Small spinach or vegetable salad
    or
    Soup (low-fat)
(b) Chicken without skin, broiled or barbecued (be aware that most barbecue sauces contain sugar)
    or
    Fish, broiled, lightly sauteed, poached, steamed, or grilled
    or
    Two slices of turkey white meat (go lightly on the gravy)
    or
    Raw vegetable salad
    or
    Spinach salad
    or
    Shrimp dish (but occasionally, not as a regular meal)
    or
    Small to medium order of pasta (also only occasionally)
(c) Brown rice, kasha, bulgur, or barley
    or
    Small baked potato, a few boiled potatoes, or yam or sweet potato
(d) Lightly cooked vegetables
(e) Apple sauce
    or
    Fresh fruit
(f) Herb tea, decaffeinated beverage, or skim milk

Break the habit of eating dessert with every meal. Eat it only occasionally. Once you break the dessert habit, you will find that you feel more alive and less inclined to be sleepy after you have eaten.

# 7

# *Fluids:*
# *The Rivers of Life*

Fluids are essential to our well-being. They play a primary role in our diet, as a way for us to ingest the nutrients we need (but also as a source of potentially harmful substances, particularly caffeine and sugar). Adequate fluid intake is essential to maintain a healthy blood volume and also for the kidneys to keep the blood filtered properly.

Fluids are particularly important for computer operators because of the physical role they play in our bodies. We tend to work in air-conditioned environments in which humidity is kept low. Direct consequences of this may include skin problems, increased vulnerability to allergic reactions, and respiratory complaints. Also, long periods sitting at the keyboard can inhibit the flow of fluids through the veins, arteries, and lymphatic channels essential to life.

So it is difficult to overemphasize the need for computer users to drink copious quantities of water and to move their bodies regularly to help maintain the necessary quantity of body fluids and to circulate those fluids throughout the body.

### Fluids and Microtrauma

Stress and microtrauma are always a major risk in long-term sitting or kneeling—indeed, in any position in which the body is fixed for extended periods. Prehistoric man suffered from cramped limbs after keeping still for hours trying to capture his lunch, but he recovered quickly because his life-style required almost continual motion. Ten thousand years later, computer users are suffering far more because they stay in fixed positions as a matter of routine for a substantial proportion of their lives.

If for no other reason, be persuaded to keep your body moving because that is the only way you are going to maintain reasonably efficient circulation in your arteries, veins, and lymphatic vessels. The arteries take the blood out from the heart to the remotest parts of the body, while the veins return this blood to the heart. The lymphatic fluids can be thought of as the body's waterways; they keep the system healthy, cleansing the tissues and flushing out the products of cellular digestion.

If you don't keep the circulation active, it becomes sluggish and you have a greater tendency to become ill or suffer an injury. Your thinking processes will also be inhibited if the brain does not get a steady, strong supply of blood. The computing analogy is failure to get good performance from a 386 system that is slowed down because it still has 8-bit circuitry on the motherboard when the electronic data processing should be flowing along 16- or 32-bit highways.

When you maintain an unnatural sitting position at the computer, you inhibit the flow of fluids through the body. Most of the body's fluid exchange occurs because of body movement, particularly joint and muscle motion. The heart is not a sufficiently large or efficient pump to circulate all the fluid necessary to maintain a healthy body. The movement of the body itself is essential to accomplish this task effectively.

So movement in the muscles and joints creates a vital additional pumping action. When the body is sedentary as it is when computing, there is a substantial lessening of fluid exchange; the pumps just cannot work properly. The metabolized products of cellular digestion tend to pool in the tissues, and so don't get flushed away readily. When we move around normally, the fluids in our body are flowing like a stream. When we are sitting down at the computer we are effectively putting dams in that flow of fluids and substantially reducing the pumping force behind them as well. This is a long-term damaging consequence quite distinct from—and in addition to—the microtrauma caused by repetitive stress.

However, there is a harmful connection. Tight muscles with restricted fluid flow are much more prone to microtrauma from repetitive stress than a healthy system. For some, just twisting around in your chair to answer the telephone can result in a painful injury when you are in such a vulnerable state.

### Digestion and Breathing

If you spend long periods sitting with poor posture, your abdomen tightens up and the flow of fluid through your digestive system is inhibited, subjecting your digestive processes to stress and malfunction.

The collapsed chest and tight belly so common among computer users has a negative effect on the quality of blood oxygen as well as on the ability of the stomach to digest food. If you don't breathe properly, your blood is not adequately oxygenated. That, in combination with lack of exercise and an inferior diet, brings on a host of problems. Here is a very easy Quick Fix to reduce these problems.

---

℞

## Quick Fix #21

Next time you feel tired and listless when working at your computer, break off work, get up, and drink a glass of cool, fresh water. Then throw back your shoulders, open up your chest, and take ten gentle deep breaths. Exhale as long as possible between the breaths. You are bound to feel better immediately—and your body will benefit the more you make this a regular habit.

---

# 8

# *Stress and Emotional Overload*

The physical and psychological stress we experience in our daily lives is becoming recognized as a major factor in a wide range of health problems. We have already seen how prolonged computer work imposes a variety of physical stresses on our bodies. Now we will examine how computers affect our psychological state. However, we must not consider the physical and the psychological health issues in isolation. Each influences the other enormously because we are such sophisticated, complex biological machines.

## Human-Machine Relationships

Stress from computer work has become a serious and complex issue because we have never before had machines that interact with us so powerfully at the emotional, psychological, and mental levels. Automobiles and other consumer goods have long been designed and marketed in ways that appeal to our emotions. Computers take this human-machine relationship into a whole new area, as illustrated by the way that computing can come to dominate the lives of some people.

Marriages have been ruined by one partner's addictive and unbalanced preoccupation with a computer. The hacker phenomenon includes thousands of predominantly young males for whom the computer has become a more comfortable, interesting, and less threatening companion than other human beings.

Our emotional relationship with our smart machines is the least-understood aspect of the impact that computing is having on both our physical and mental well-being. But it is important to consider it fully when developing your strategies for happy, healthy computing.

## The Physical and Emotional Links

The physical stresses that we impose on our bodies when computing can have serious adverse emotional consequences as well. A habitually tight body subjected to prolonged periods of tension may develop both structural and emotional problems when the stress is continually beyond tolerance levels.

If you learn to relax your body and have healthy work habits, you will find that many emotional work tensions decrease. You will be better able to cope with stress that may be aggravated by conditions in

---

℞

# Quick Fix #22

You may be able to reduce stress and frustration significantly without the expense of buying new equipment. For example, experiment with the software controls that vary the speed of the cursor movement in many applications programs. Write macro programs, if they do not exist already in your program, to eliminate altogether the most frustrating sequences of keyboard instructions that you do regularly.

Experiment with programs—many available as shareware— that vary the blinking rate, size, and other characteristics of the cursor, the point on the screen that you focus on most. Just as you vary your working posture in your chair, you can use software to run through the range of possible variations in how the computer functions. There are lots of such tricks.

your environment, such as the noise and light levels and distractions from colleagues.

Your hardware and software may be significant stressors. A database or word processor that is difficult to use can make you very tense. Not being taught properly can build up the stress levels enormously, because you may never feel fully comfortable and in control of a particular applications program, a specific computer task, or just computing generally.

Deficient hardware can be infuriating, and anger, especially suppressed anger, is at the root of many headaches and other health problems. Poorly placed keys or a keyboard without the tactile response with which you are most comfortable can generate a great deal of stress very quickly.

You need to be comfortable and at ease with your equipment, so give thought to changing something like a keyboard or a mouse that just does not fit your style of working.

## Make the Most of the Easiest Tasks

Among the most tiring, demanding, and otherwise stressful computer tasks is having to key in a lot of data. It is made even worse if the text or numbers are detailed and must be captured accurately. So you need to make the most of the time you inevitably spend on other, less demanding computer tasks.

When editing, spell-checking, or brainstorming, lean back and relax because these are probably activities that do not require you to be hunched over the keyboard constantly referring to papers. Everything is happening on the screen and probably not requiring intensive inputting, just the occasional hitting of a few keys or a mouse movement to make changes. You could also perform these tasks standing up.

You can put the keyboard on your lap, or put it and the mouse on a simple lap tray. Adjust the line spacing of the text on the display to make it easier to read—just setting the whole text for double or triple spacing can transform the appearance of a word processing document and make it easier to work with.

Perhaps change the screen colors also to fit your mood. Or switch into the graphics mode that many word processors now support. It may make the text on the screen and the cursor much larger, so you may be able to take off your reading glasses, lean back, and give your eyes a change of scenery also. You may benefit from switching occasionally—or permanently—to a large-type word processor, such as Ken Skier's classic Eye Relief. If you are copying large or complex text or figures, consider dictating them to yourself on a recorder/transcriber.

## Don't Get Angry With Your Computer

Please take very seriously the need to establish a comfortable and amicable relationship with your computer. It is not a funky concept, but is at least as important for your physical health and emotional well-being as having good relationships with your human work associates.

Hostility—even to the point of outright violence—has featured in our relationships with machines since the Industrial Revolution in the eighteenth century. Now hostility characterizes the relationships many of us have with the new smart machines of the twentieth century's Information Revolution.

This hostility and other negative feelings experienced by millions who have had their working lives transformed by computer technology lie at the root of many physical health problems. The pain in your head, your back, your neck, or your eyes may well be caused, at least in part, by bad management on the part of your superiors, conflict with your colleagues, dissatisfaction with your working situation, defects in your working environment, or a sense of loss of control and vulnerability because of problems with your hardware or software.

We have already emphasized how interdependent all the physical elements of our bodies are. The physical well-being of our bodies is also dependent on our mental and emotional states. Many of us who use computers intensively have very negative feelings about them that we may not be able to express clearly, even if we recognize them at all. This was demonstrated graphically by a group of clerical workers surveyed by Shoshana Zuboff when researching her classic book *In the Age of the Smart Machine: The Future of Work & Power* (New York: Basic Books, 1988). These workers drew pictures that spoke more powerfully than any words they expressed of the emotional conflicts they experienced when interfacing with computers.

# Expensive Stress

The Congressional Office of Technology Assessment (OTA) has warned that stress-related illness could be costing American businesses $75 billion a year. The problem is aggravated by the pressures imposed when both the pace and nature of work is dictated by computerization.

Computers are dehumanizing work, breaking it up into specific, routine, and often boring tasks. Those who just do limited routine work, such as data entry, feel suppressed anger and frustration, accentuated by their resentment at being controlled by machines. About a third of all U.S. clerical workers are now monitored by computer to some extent. Increasingly, the computer measures and records how many times they hit the keys, how many errors they make, and when and how often they take breaks to go to the rest room or the watercooler.

In some countries—notably Germany and Sweden—workers have openly expressed their strong feelings about this dehumanizing situation. They have demanded work breaks, rotation of jobs, and measures to ease the sensations of loneliness and isolation that characterize many computerized offices.

American computer operators have been less militant, at least until recently, but obviously their feelings are just as strong. When the anger and resentment caused by emotional and psychological stresses are suppressed, they inevitably become expressed in some other way. One consequence is the increase of localized "epidemics" of physical injuries related to computer work. When one person in a group is diagnosed with carpal tunnel syndrome, eyestrain, or some other definable physical problem, a high proportion of other members of the group soon display similar confirmed symptoms.

# Human Issues Are Paramount

The negative results of introducing computers to the workplace become most serious in organizations and working environments that pay too little attention to human issues and too much to the productivity improvements that computers appear to offer. There are thousands of offices around the world where the management has deliberately isolated employees from contact with each other while they are working. This has been seen as an integral part of the changes necessary in the work environment to achieve the productivity required to give the appropriate payback from expensive computerization.

As computers have been introduced as tools for workers to use, they have been cast also as Big Brother machines to monitor productivity and work quality. The OTA warned back in 1987 about the dangers of "electronic sweatshops" in which the supervisor is not human, but an "unwinking computer taskmaster." Over 20 million people in the United States alone now experience a situation in which a computer, instead of a human supervisor, is constantly looking over their shoulders, checking on what they are doing.

Not surprisingly, this is a dehumanizing, demotivating situation that increases stress and negative attitudes toward work generally—and toward computers in particular. We resent these smart machines as we would a human supervisor who does not extend to us the trust to do our jobs as well as we are able. Our self-esteem takes a knock, we become resentful, and we develop a hostility, the obvious target of which is the computer.

Such a situation compounds the stress already generated by protracted periods of intensive work at a computer. In *In the Age of the Smart Machine*, Shoshana Zuboff describes how a group of clerical workers in her study reacted to the introduction of computerization by withdrawing into the confines of their individual body spaces. They became introverted in their attitudes, so, as happens to most of us when we feel sorry for ourselves, their attention focused on their physical discomfort. They became more conscious of these discomforts and inevitably blamed them on the catalyst for their emotional distress—the computers.

This is a vicious cycle that anyone who manages computer operators—or, equally important, those of us who manage ourselves—must consider just as carefully as the physical ergonomic qualities of the chair in which we sit or the clarity of the screen at which we look. Medical science is still woefully ignorant of how the mind affects the body, but there is universal agreement that it has a very powerful influence over the body's physical well-being. If you are unhappy and stressed using a computer, you greatly increase the chances that you will perceive the computer as a source of physical distress.

We don't even need to get into a discussion of the differences between pain or other symptoms that are caused by a tangible injury or infection and those that may arise from mental and emotional triggers. If it hurts, it hurts, no matter what the cause. If your distress is genuine and you blame the computer, both you and your employer, if you have one, need to take remedial action.

## Identify the Antagonists

Often the symptoms are there but we do not recognize the causes—the irritants or antagonists. There are many things wrong with our modern life-styles, so it can be very difficult for us to identify why we are not as happy and do not feel physically as well as we should. When Shoshana Zuboff asked the clerical workers she was studying to draw pictures of how they felt about their jobs before and after they were converted to a new computer system, the resulting drawings showed a remarkable consistency of negative emotional reactions. The largest group of pictures showed that the workers perceived that their bodies had changed as a direct result of the introduction of computers. These changes included hair loss; impaired eyesight; contortion of facial muscles; radical decrease in bodily dimensions; rigidification of the torso, arms, and faces; inability to speak or hear; immobility; and headaches.

In *In the Age of the Smart Machine,* Zuboff states:

> The clerks portrayed themselves as chained to desks, surrounded by bottles of aspirin, dressed in prison stripes, outfitted with blinders, closely observed by their supervisors, surrounded by walls, enclosed without sunlight or food, bleary-eyed with fatigue, solitary, frowning, and blank—without a face.

The pressure and negative emotional feelings experienced by those hostile to their computing work can cause severe mental stress and also lead to a host of physical problems. The symptoms and illnesses that the clerks displayed in their drawings of how they perceived themselves are now occurring in epidemic proportions in offices everywhere.

## The Dangers of Isolation and Repetition

People are being forced to work in isolation because computers reduce—often almost eliminate—the need and opportunity for direct human communication. People, like laboratory rats, display extreme stress and aberrant behavior when confined for long periods in isolation.

Although computing has been hailed as eliminating many boring, repetitive tasks, for many clerical workers it has also introduced monotony and repetition, the stress of which is compounded by the need to maintain close attention to avoid inputting errors, but without the mental stimuli that can make such attention healthy or even tolerable. You do not get nearly as stressed having to concentrate on something that is interesting and satisfying.

This is not a new phenomenon peculiar to computer technology. Way back in 1960, when automation and mechanization were first starting to gain ground in the office environment, the International Labor Organization (ILO) published the results of a major study that showed the then-new forms of mechanical office automation were generating nervous tension that posed a greater threat than the physical exertion the machines were designed to reduce.

The ILO noted that the consequences of the strain of having to pay close attention to repetitive work included mental and nervous disorders, emotional disturbances, irritability, nervousness, hypersensitivity, insomnia, various functional disturbances, headaches, digestive disorders, heart troubles, states of depression, and many more.

These were the consequences identified three decades ago during the interim stage of office automation—electric typewriters, adding machines, and the like. The move to computers—the electronic phase of office automation—in the last ten years has taken place far more rapidly and represents far greater changes in work practices, so the human consequences are much greater also.

## Keeping in Touch With Reality

A sense of losing touch with reality is among the emotional and psychological results of working with computers rather than carrying out tasks through traditional, more physical methods. Our work becomes dominated by abstract rather than tangible things because computing changes three-dimensional reality into two-dimensional digital symbols. Researchers have determined that this generates sensations of loss of control and consequent feelings of vulnerability among many computer operators.

An important element in the hacker phenomenon is that some computing enthusiasts are more comfortable interfacing with computers than other humans. They find the two-dimensional digital environment less emotionally demanding than coping with normal multidimensional human interactions. So, for thousands of youngsters, computers have provided an escape from the traumas of teenage life.

On a more positive note, those who can blend computers successfully into their lives find it an enriching and enjoyable experience. The ability of the smart machines to take over demanding, repetitive tasks and extend our human mental capabilities is an invaluable resource. *Computing can offer many rewards and even reduce stress and negative emotions.*

## Achieve a Positive Computing Environment and Attitude

Unfortunately, we miss the payoff, the rewards of computer technology, when we allow them to create a discomforting, unfriendly environment.

The computing environment is particularly unwelcoming to those of us who did not grow up with this technology or who find it difficult to understand. Studies of students and professional people indicate that about a third display symptoms of "computerphobia," or extreme anxiety and nervousness about using computers. Many of us find computers intimidating, and our performance and states of mental and physical health when we use them are greatly influenced by such attitudes.

The attitude we have toward our work can be the key to many computing-related health problems. It may influence that sense of inner energy that is so important to all of us and have tangible effects on stress levels and resultant physical symptoms.

Negative work attitudes can be detrimental to body posture, because our attitude and how we feel about ourselves and other things in our lives are expressed in our body language. Attitude also affects breathing. It can manifest itself in unconscious jaw clenching, which an hour or two later may result in a headache. For your health's sake, you need to take definite action to reduce those things which contribute to a negative attitude toward computer work and develop those that are positive.

## Stressful Software

Although most of the blame for stress and negative attitudes in the workplace is imputed to hardware, furniture, and other physical factors, inferior software contributes much to these problems also.

You need to be careful in your selection of software so that you relate well to a computer and are comfortable using it. Complex, poorly written software with inadequate documentation or on-line help facilities and other defects can make you very uptight, because your knowledge of it is limited and you're constantly in an antagonistic relationship with something you feel you cannot control.

Of course, a similar situation can arise with good software if you do not allocate the time to learn it properly. Much computer frustration— as well as loss of productivity—comes from not reading the manuals or practicing the tutorials that come with the program disks!

## Preserve Your Humanity

Fundamental to creating a positive work attitude is retaining one's sense of humanity, individualism, and self-worth. You must preserve your humanity when you are computing and not become dominated by the smart machine, even if you are stimulated and fascinated by it. Only by maintaining an awareness of yourself will you allow your breathing to be full and relaxed and maintain a natural, balanced posture that protects your body and ensures that it functions in an efficient and healthy way.

Preserve your humanity and sense of self or you will stop monitoring your body's welfare and so increase its exposure to harm. In our natural mental states we function as we are designed to and continually monitor the levels of pleasure and pain we are experiencing. We are genetically programmed to move toward pleasure and away from pain. If this process is changed because we become disconnected from ourselves and no longer in direct tune with our humanity, we become very prone to injury from such unconscious actions as adopting a distorted, fixed posture without realizing it.

Our minds may be so preoccupied with the first machines capable of totally absorbing our attention and establishing the most intimate intellectual relationships with us that we lose the sense of our physical humanity to the point of shutting off some of the body's natural monitoring systems. We risk our bodies becoming rather like taxis that bring our minds to work. Computing can be so absorbing, so demanding, that our bodies can easily become just the vehicles that deliver our brains to the computer so that we can wiggle our fingers and have this interaction with the dominating, addictive, ever-challenging machine.

This phenomenon raises a number of important and complex issues, some of which appear incomprehensible to computer professionals who are confident, because of their expertise, when they interact with smart machines. Many of the managers and decision makers who control the choice of hardware and software and who manage computing activities cannot relate to the frustration and feelings of being threatened that many of us who are not as well trained, expert, or confident experience at the keyboard.

Our sense of loss of control is heightened when we have to run programs that are not user-friendly, and we can become particularly stressed when something goes wrong and we are made even more aware of our computing limitations. Zuboff found a manifestation of this when she was doing research in a timber processing plant where operators were particularly hostile to the computer and the automatic production control system. They had mounted a large ax on the wall of the control room, with a sign underneath reading: IN CASE OF COMPUTER FAILURE, USE FIRE AXE.

That left no doubt of the workers' hostility toward their computers. The smart machines had become adversaries, and adversarial relationships are not healthy.

"Must the new electronic milieu engender a world in which individuals have lost control over their daily work lives?" Zuboff asks.

The answer is no. If your work environment is controlled by managers insensitive to these vital human issues relating to computer work, you may need to take firm, positive action to seek improvements. Press for the removal of the partitions that isolate you from visual and auditory contact with your fellow workers and so heighten the intensity of the human–machine interaction. Demand regular work breaks, which are essential for physical health and also to mental and emotional well-being among computer operators. You need to get away from the machine and back into contact with the real world at frequent intervals, say every 60–90 minutes, if you are going to be a reasonably happy as well as productive computer operator. It is in the interest of employers also to tackle these problems. The message is clear. Unhappy, hostile, stressed-out workers do not generate good, long-term, bottom-line results for their employers, even if shallow, short-term, time-and-motion studies indicate otherwise.

---

℞

# Quick Fix #23

Make the most of all your breaks to get emotional as well as physical refreshment. Over lunch or when visiting the watercooler or rest room, make a conscious effort to communicate with colleagues. Make, not avoid, the eye contacts, the exchange of verbal pleasantries, the few minutes of gossip, and other social interchanges that used to permeate a normal office working day but now, since the computer has become so dominant, may be confined largely to the break periods.

---

We owe it ourselves to fight back at trends to dehumanize our working environment. We need, some of us more than others, to personalize our work spaces. We need the photographs of our children or other loved ones, the low-tech clippings or Post-it notes to jog our memories of personal things needing our attention in those parts of our lives not dominated by the computer. Maybe we like to keep our pens and pencils in an old chipped mug, or have a wood carving or bunch of flowers on our desk. Computerization has tended to bring with it a trend to uniformity and undue emphasis on functional efficiency in workplaces, subjugating individual expression to a perceived inferior role.

Some of the unhappiest, most stressed, and frustrated workers are those in offices where the machines and the interior decorators impose an environment. Some of the happiest, least stressed computer users have blended their high-tech machines into workplaces that express their own personalities, creating environments that have evolved and reflect the humans in them rather than being dominated by the needs of their machines.

If you are your own boss, or work mainly at home, then you have control over your computing environment and should use this power to create a place where stress is minimized and positive emotional and mental stimulation enhanced. Don't shut yourself away in a corner, following traditional conventions that work should be relegated to second-class areas of a home, while entertaining, eating, and other activities take pride of place in the allocation of domestic resources. If you are spending many hours generating the income that sustains the home, you are more than entitled to do your work in the prime part of the home.

That could be the room with the view, or with the space for you to work comfortably with the least stress and the maximum enjoyment. Decorate it to please yourself, with colors, pictures, ornaments, and furniture that delight your eye and give you pleasure.

Don't be conned by convention into installing your system on a sterile, contemporary office desk. A PC can function very well when housed in a traditional rolltop desk or placed on an antique table. Computers have removed many of the sensory pleasures of working with tools and materials. Some writers still cannot create unless there is a physical sensation of their thoughts flowing through their bodies and being turned into words laid down by hand movements of pen or pencil across the surface of a sheet of paper. Others have adapted to the new technology and find it far more satisfactory to have the speed and flexibility of hitting a keyboard and manipulating their creative efforts on a screen display. But all of us can still benefit from stimulating our physical senses and not being confined to an unnatural—if more efficient—electronic working environment.

So don't deprive yourself of sensory pleasure when working at your computer. Touching a work surface of warm, textured old wood, having flowers in a bowl near your keyboard, or a table fountain tinkling nearby, provide the sensory stimulation or relaxation that can add much to one's sense of reality when working with dehumanizing high-tech equipment and abstract, two-dimensional data. This obviously may be more important when the computing task is repetitive and intellectually undemanding, but you also need to keep in touch with reality when your attitude toward the computer is entirely positive and it is helping you to achieve your dreams, for example when you are writing the great American novel.

Music can be a particularly effective influence on emotional work states. In some companies the tempo of background music is actually programmed to counter increasing worker fatigue toward the end of the day or the shift. But as well as providing a positive stimulus, music can also have negative, stressful effects, sometimes without listeners' being aware of the fact. A study at Penn State University indicated that people do not relax to music they do not like, and that even "easy listening" music can generate stress in those who do not enjoy it.

Some heavy rock and other music with a strong beat can build up tension. Other tempos and frequencies can have a marked calming effect. We still know very little about how music and other auditory stimuli affect our emotions in general and the physical functioning of the brain in particular.

The brain generates waves of energy in distinctive states. These include the alpha state, when we are at our most relaxed and probably functioning most efficiently for creative tasks; the normal beta state of wakefulness, when we are most alert; the theta state at the verge of sleep, when we are very receptive to learning and remembering; and the deep sleep of the delta state. Shift workers are particularly vulnerable to physical and emotional stress when the natural rhythm of these brain patterns is disrupted.

Shift workers particularly may benefit from current research into variations in both light and sound to alter these states in which visual and audio cues are used to reduce work stress and increase productivity. The research is controversial, but sufficiently well founded for you to pay special attention to both the desirable and, perhaps, undesirable effects on your mental and emotional states caused by music and other noise.

Individuals react very differently to various types of music, so it may be impossible to have music playing that will be beneficial to everyone in the same work space. What is soothing or stimulating to some people may be distracting or irritating to others. There are variations also in preferred volume levels. Music that seems at the correct volume for some may be distressingly loud for others.

There are considerable dangers inherent in using earphones for prolonged periods to try to create your own musical environment. They increase the sense of isolation, can be stressful, and sometimes allow the volume to creep up to a level that can damage your hearing.

# 9

# Making Your Chair and Desk Fit You

The most important items of computer hardware as far as comfort and health are concerned are your chair and desk, especially the chair. If your work and your life involve protracted periods sitting down, get yourself a good chair as a high health priority. However fit and tough you are, remember that no human being has yet been born who can sit in the best chair that has ever been made and work for two hours at a computer without stressing the body in ways that can injure it over a longer period of time.

If you are an employee and your employer will not provide you with a chair that will adjust satisfactorily to your physique and workstation, buy one yourself. You may set the lead in your organization for better seating to become the priority that it should.

If you are self-employed or otherwise do a lot of computing at home, budget for a good chair, even if you can only afford to buy it on credit. Every monthly installment is bound to be cheaper than treatment later to remedy the ravages than can be caused by an inferior chair. Claim—and if necessary fight for—tax relief for the chair and desk you need to earn a living, or which is recommended by your doctor or therapist for health reasons.

## Sitting Is Dangerous

Inferior chairs, coupled with the incorrect ways in which we sit, cause more industrial and personal injuries in the United States and other Western developed countries than autos, handguns, and factory machinery combined. Asian, African, and Oriental societies have been substantially less at risk from chairs because their cultural heritages encourage them to squat, kneel, or sit on the floor. Now, with the pervasive spread of contemporary Western cultures, millions of people are sitting and hurting themselves all over the world.

The cost to American business of having its workers sit down— particularly its computer operators—is enormous. The National Insurance Council estimates that over 100 million workdays are lost each year and there is a $20 billion annual cost in losses attributable to absenteeism as a result of back injuries. A high proportion of back problems stem from incorrect sitting. It is a high probability that any

℞

# Quick Fix #24

Check to make sure that you are following these basic rules on posture at the keyboard:

- Sit upright, arching your lower back and with your head up and balanced naturally over your shoulders. Experiment with a small cushion in the lumbar region of the small of your back to help you maintain this posture.
- Place your feet flat on the floor, with your knees lower than your buttocks. Most of your weight should be on the buttocks—definitely not pinching the nerves and restricting blood flow behind your thighs or knees.
- Have your elbows almost at right angles, not resting on the chair arms, and with a gentle downward slope from your elbows to your fingers on the keyboard.
- Adjust your chair to adopt this position relative to your workstation. If doing so makes it impossible for your feet to rest flat on the floor, use a footrest. If it is not possible to achieve this position at all, you will need to modify or change the chair and/or the workstation. One quick fix that may be enough is to add a keyboard drawer below the work surface to lower the keyboard sufficiently.

heavy computer user with back pain, particularly lower-back pain, has an inferior chair.

Only the common cold causes more lost productivity in the United States than injured backs. But that's only the tip of the iceberg. When you add in medical care, drugs, the purchase of products claiming to ease the suffering, and legal awards, our bad backs cost the country over $80 billion a year, according to Insurance Council estimates.

The more you probe the statistics, the more amazing it seems that we tolerate such enormous quantities of unnecessary pain, suffering, and expense from unhealthy backs. The American Academy of Orthopedic Surgeons estimates that at least $3 billion is spent on tests and treatment just for lumbar disk disorders—one small part of a much bigger problem universally agreed to stem mainly from sitting improperly.

Over 75 percent of us perform most of our tasks at work while sitting down. Our culture has preserved the status symbolism surrounding chairs and so ensures that many managers are sitting more dangerously than the workers for whom they are responsible! Appearance and prestige in furniture often triumph over ergonomics. In the business world, some of the most expensive and ergonomically least satisfactory chairs and desks are to be found in executive offices.

In enlightened organizations, the computer operators have high-tech furniture to go with their high-tech machines. Where chairs are properly recognized for their contribution to bottom-line productivity from seated workers, productivity and health both get a boost.

## Expert Advice on Good Seating

Real expertise in the special seating needs of computer users is hard to find. To get the best advice available we went to an expert who has a passionate interest in sitting correctly because he understands the impact it can have on all aspects of health.

"Headaches, backaches, and many other health problems are a direct result of sitting incorrectly," says Hector Serber, president of the American Ergonomics Corporation. Serber has devoted many years seeking solutions to seating problems, including his own as a sufferer from lower-back pain.

He agrees with our message in this book that we interrupt the natural balance and movement of the body when we sit down. Bending at the hip and knee joints imposes unnatural forces of tension, pressure, and compression on the musculoskeletal system, and also restricts essential fluid flow through the body and inhibits full inhaling and exhaling when we breathe.

"We think of sitting as being safe, relaxing, and restful, but extensive scientific research shows the opposite is usually the case," says Serber. "Sitting down increases internal lumbar disk pressure by 35 percent compared to standing. Then leaning forward by 40 degrees—the posture adopted by some computer users when they are concentrating hard—can increase compression at points in the lumbar joints to nearly 500 pounds. That is the point at which these joints would rupture, if their supporting musculature was not taking the strain."

## Your Chair Should Protect—Not Hurt—Your Body

As a computer user, you should realize that your chair is far more than just a support for the body. Your chair is your first line of defense to protect your body from the abuse of sitting (see Figure 5).

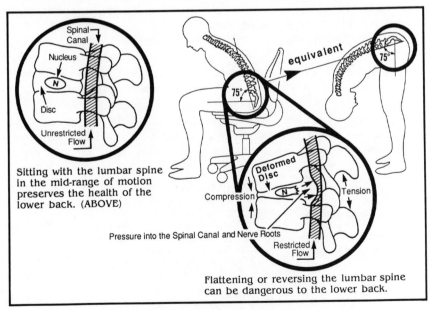

**Figure 5.** Abuse the body takes from sitting.

Just being comfortable and sitting ergonomically correctly when you stay in one position for a long time is not enough. In fact, it can be positively harmful to be too comfortable because you are likely then to stay in that one position virtually all the time. It may even be healthier to sit in an uncomfortable chair in which you are forced to keep changing positions (as long as you can maintain the natural shape of the lumbar spine) than in one that encourages you to remain static so that joints and muscles become fixed and unmoving.

So, when you are seeking the chair that is ideal for you, look for mobility as much as comfort. That search steers many of us at one time or another to consider the backless kneeling seat, with one pad for our rumps and another placed forward and at an angle on which we rest our knees. Although beneficial in many respects, even the best kneeling chairs fall down in one important respect. The sustained pressure put on your knee joints by these chairs eventually can create serious microtrauma if you use one for long-term, intensive work.

So if you use a kneeling chair, sometimes shift positions so that your weight is alternately on one knee at a time, with the foot of the other leg resting on the floor. Do not sit for long, intensive periods with both knees under continuous compression, because that risks cumulative trauma to the joint structures.

Also try to alternate between using the kneeling chair and sitting in another providing back support. Kneeling helps to preserve the natural curves of the spine and keeps the head and arms in balance if you are working in an erect position. However, many deskbound tasks, including computing, encourage one to adopt a slightly reclined position, and with intensive work, a chair with a back and shin rest (and your feet on the floor) can deal more effectively with this problem.

However, it is beneficial to your body to change position for some computing tasks and spend a period leaning back and relaxing. Most sitting chairs make this very difficult. Your butt tends to slide forward without knee or foot support to keep you in place, forcing your lower back into a slouched position.

### Watch the Angles

For healthy sitting, it is critical to have the least stressful angles at the points of the body that have to bend. The National Aeronautics and Space Administration found that an angle of 135 degrees between the trunk of your upper body and your thighs and an approximately 90-degree angle at the knees come naturally to weightless astronauts. But unless you are using your computer in space, gravity is working against you and you are inhibited from achieving these desirable natural angles because of the need to support your weight and because of the design of your chair (see Figure 6).

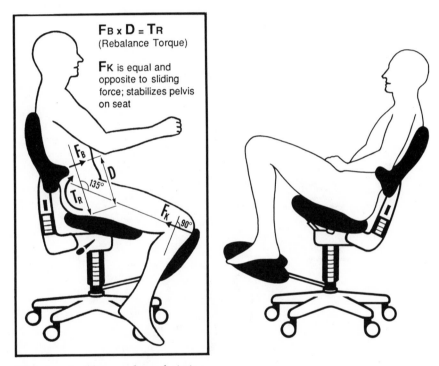

$$F_B \times D = T_R$$
(Rebalance Torque)

$F_K$ is equal and opposite to sliding force; stabilizes pelvis on seat

**Figure 6.** The angles of sitting.

You need a chair that spreads the load at your back, has an angled seat to maintain even and acceptable loads on the buttocks and thighs, and provides a knee rest for further support. A seat pad that swivels around the horizontal axis is an added benefit to cope with gravity's forces and realign your spine as you change position at your workstation. In some positions you will put more weight on the forward edge of the

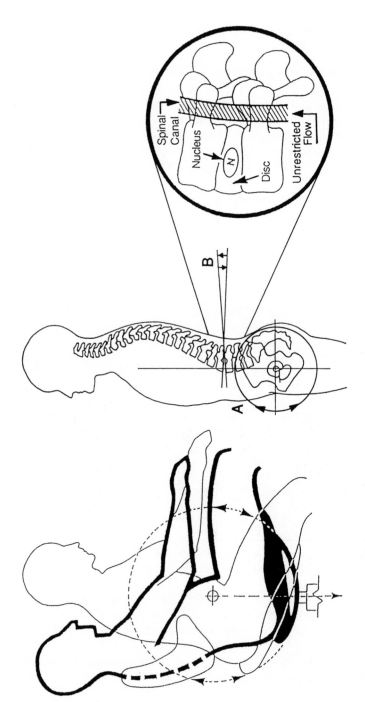

**Figure 7.** Hector Serber's continuous balance seat.

seat behind your knees; in other positions the weight will be more to the rear.

"The resistance of a fixed seat to an active body results in increased tension along the posterior line of musculature, especially in the thighs, buttocks, and lumbar spine," says Hector Serber. "When using a computer, these muscular systems must contract for long periods above the fatigue level, traumatizing the whole musculoskeletal system surrounding those areas. Seats should swivel from the body's center so that they enable the seated body to come close to achieving the balance and natural beneficial movements that are derived from walking."

His point is illustrated in Figure 7.

When we walk, there is a constant rotating and balancing motion. The pelvis balances the weight of the trunk in conjunction with rotating the hip joints. A normal chair with a fixed seat pad restricts this natural functional integration of the body's components. The body becomes out of balance, so there are further unnatural stresses invoked just to stay in the chair. That adds up to a double whammy—you are using excess muscular effort to maintain an unnatural position, while also preventing the natural muscle and joint movements that help to maintain muscle tone and promote the flow of blood and spinal fluid.

## Preserve Your Overall Health

A particular design defect to watch out for, even in chairs that do have movable seat pads, is one that elevates your knees and positions your thighs at the wrong angle. Your back, neck, and overall health will benefit if your knees are slightly lower than your buttocks. You may be able to achieve that by adjusting the height of the chair from the floor or by putting a wedge-shaped piece of dense foam rubber on top of the seat cushion (with the thick end of the wedge at the back of the seat).

This forward angle, with the knees lower than the buttocks, may be easier to maintain with some kind of foot support. But don't use one that raises your feet so high that the knees are above the buttocks. Some computer users and typists swear they are more comfortable with their feet propped up on a pile of telephone directories, but that could well be because they have bad chairs that press hard on the back of the thighs behind the knees, causing restricted blood flow and cramps. A footrest may ease that pressure, but if it raises the knees too high, it may cause other long-term problems because that destabilizes the lower back and forces the upper body to lean forward.

It is amazing how those of us who use computers—and those who employ us to operate them—are prepared to spend so much on expensive hardware and software, but then cut costs to the bone on the vital chair! Think of your chair as an integral part of your computer system—so important that when you need to upgrade your system you may well find that it enhances your productivity more to buy a new chair than a larger hard disk or expanded memory.

To get all the desirable seating features, you may need two or three good chairs, alternating between them when computing for extended periods. Very few chairs come even close to being ideal for sustained

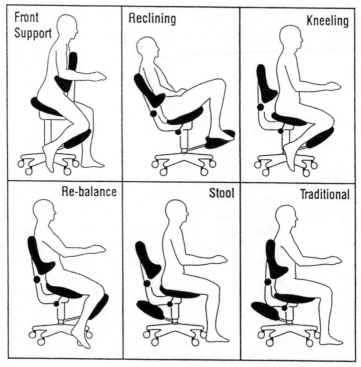

**Figure** 8. The Ergomax by Hector Serber, showing various positions.

computer usage. The Ergomax invented and patented by Hector Serber is a rare example (see Figure 8). It is not cheap at around $1,000, but treatments for an injured back can prove much more expensive. Indeed, whatever you spend on an ergonomically superior chair could be the most cost-effective investment in your system.

---

℞

## Quick Fix #25

Test your seating to find out if it is a health hazard, and identify what improvements you need to make. Go through the text and illustrations in this section, noting whether your chair—or the one you intend to buy—meets the important requirements we recommend. If it does not, take an ergonomically correct chair into your life, adjust it to fit you and your workstation, and you could achieve significant improvements in your health.

---

The pictures of the Ergomax in this chapter provide benchmarks for the desirable characteristics in a computer user's chair. The University of Iowa Medical Center's Physical Therapy Research Department (in a study done for the American Ergonomics Corporation) found that the front support of the Ergomax eliminates over 50 percent of the muscle tension in the lower back normally associated with traditional postures.

Dr. Arthur White, medical director of St. Mary's Spine Center in San Francisco, who looks after back problems among the 49ers football team, says the Ergomax is the most innovative back chair in the world. One user was so enthusiastic that he had the chair and stool combination fitted to his bass boat so that he could be as comfortable fishing as he was at his desk!

The two main sitting postures computer users need to adopt are illustrated in Figure 9.

If you want more information about the Ergomax, the American Ergonomics Corporation is at 200 Gate Five Road, Sausalito, California 94965 (415/332-5635).

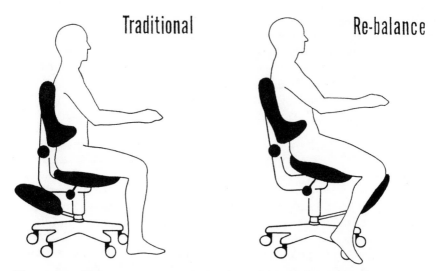

Figure   9. The two main sitting postures for the computer user in the
Ergomax.

## Alternative Ways to Ease Chair Pain

If you cannot invest in an ergonomically good chair, or your
employer will not provide one, don't despair. There are ways of
achieving at least some improvement to a standard desk and chair to
make inferior equipment kinder to your body.

You can modify any chair to some extent with cushions or sections
of wedged plastic foam. Hold them in place with duct tape and put a
loose cover over the chair if appearance is less critical than comfort.

If you cannot raise a chair high enough because it does not have
sufficient adjustment, try mounting it on larger casters. Or take off the
existing casters, screw a square or circle of thick wood to the feet of the
chair, and then refasten the casters to the underside of the wood. Use
several pieces of wood to achieve the necessary added height. Or put
your chair on a thick sheet of wood to adjust the height appropriately.

Much can be done to improve seating simply by changing the way
you sit, and also, of course, by taking any opportunity you can to relax
or work in a standing position and to walk around.

All computer users—even those sitting in expensive chairs—need to practice healthy work habits. Just keep in mind how the body was designed to be used and consequently how it should interface in a healthy way with computers.

Go back to Quick Fix #24 at the start of this chapter and review the general points about posture. Then you should enjoy immediate benefits from achieving a proper sitting posture—one in which the hands, arms, and head in particular are in positions relative to each other that preserve bodily functional integration.

Don't sit still for hours on end—even in the best chair. The importance of regular movement cannot be overemphasized. Stress and microtrauma are always inherent in long-term sitting or kneeling—indeed, in any fixed position for extended periods.

Change position regularly. Even in the most comfortable chair, change the position you work in at frequent intervals, and use the exercises that we recommend. This combination will increase your productivity and substantially reduce the consequences of accumulated stress that are inherent in long-term computer use.

## What About Your Desk?

Although the desk is the largest component of a computer workstation, it need not be expensive, sophisticated, or "high tech" to contribute to your good health.

Follow the advice on chairs and sitting and make your desk or other working surface conform to those requirements. Make your desk fit you, do not adapt yourself and your posture to conform to this dumb piece of furniture!

If you have adjusted your chair correctly and still need to alter your desk height, there are various alternatives to consider. It is not difficult to raise the height of a desk—or of the keyboard, if that is the problem. Wooden blocks under the legs of the desk, or a piece of wood planking or foam rubber under the keyboard and mouse pad, are usually quick and easy fixes.

However, because most desks are designed for paper work, you usually need to make the work surface lower so that there is that natural slightly downward slope from the elbows to the fingers that so effectively reduces repetitive stress injuries to the wrist and hand. Perhaps you can cut off pieces from the legs of the desk, or raise your chair still higher. Consider also installing a keyboard drawer under the desk to achieve the correct operating height—and to free more desk space when not computing. Don't forget to have a drawer large enough for mouse operation also; even if you don't use a mouse now, you probably will in the future.

Consider whether you need a desk at all. Most of them are overpriced and lack flexibility. You may be more comfortable and efficient with a workstation made of two small filing cabinets supporting a door laid flat as the work surface. The height of the surface can be varied with blocks on top of the cabinets to support the door.

## The Adjustable Workstation

Particular problems arise when two or more people of different size have to use the same workstation, as in shift work or when sharing hardware. Then there may be a need for both chair and work surface to vary in height. There are proprietary workstation units that make this possible with various mechanical systems that move the table section up and down, but they tend to be expensive. The best option for all computer users is to have a fully adjustable workstation that changes conveniently to accommodate any sitting position and rises high enough so that you can also work standing up.

One such unit, designed by Colin Haynes and shown in Figure 10, won an award at the Oregon Wood Products Exposition in 1990. A unique feature is its suitability for disabled people confined to wheelchairs or beds. Both monitor and keyboard drawer move up or down to any height at the turn of a handle.

The whole computing system—central processor, monitor, keyboard, printer, modem, reading lights, floppy disks and documents, and other ancillaries are contained in a single mobile unit. So this workstation can be moved from room to room, or brought out from a closet to turn any room immediately into a fully functioning office. It will also roll over a bed or a reclining chair for those who need or prefer to do their computing lying down.

The design makes it almost impossible for anyone to get close enough to the monitor to risk damage from electromagnetic radiation. There are a variety of holders and book rests to help handle docu-

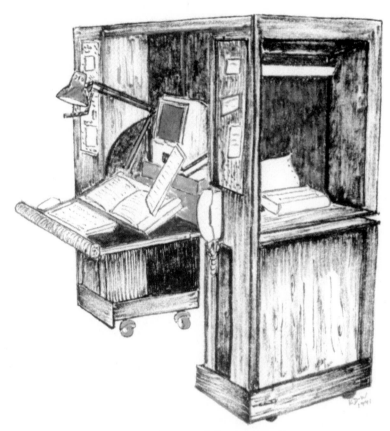

**Figure 10.** An accommodating mobile workstation.

ments, software manuals, and other paper work efficiently. Curtains conceal the equipment and convert the workstation into a discreet piece of furniture when it is not being used. The curtains also adjust to control ambient light levels and reflections affecting the monitor display.

The central processing unit—with its often noisy fan and disk drives—is housed vertically in a ventilated compartment where it is out of earshot but still within easy reach.

This workstation demonstrates what can be achieved to create a fully flexible, practical, and healthy computing environment. It can be built for a materials cost of under $200 by anyone reasonably competent with a saw, drill, and screwdriver. Use it for inspiration—building your own ideal computing environment can be as creative and challenging as actually using the computer.

If you'd like more details about this and other adjustable desks, send a stamped, addressed envelope marked "DESK" to Colin Haynes at 1257 Siskiyou Boulevard, Suite 179, Ashland, OR 97520.

# 10

# If You Manage People Who Use Computers

Computer-related health problems are a human resources issue that will not go away. At the start of 1991, efforts had been made in over thirty American states to create legislation that would compel employers to do such things as initiate programs to train their computer operators on basic health matters related to their work, provide furniture that would adjust to accommodate different sizes of operators, and mandate regular breaks away from the screen.

In some places there is lobbying for stronger measures, particularly regarding electromagnetic emissions from monitors. But, generally, the proposals have been modest in the demands they make on the business community, with generous time allowances before they come into effect.

Yet everywhere business interests have mounted strong counter-lobbies and we have started to see—particularly from computer industry interests—public relations efforts uncomfortably close to those the tobacco industry pioneered to confuse the public and protect its interests.

New York's Suffolk County had made a breakthrough in 1988 with laws imposing modest basic requirements on workstations. Local business interests—with national behind-the-scenes support—were successful in reversing this legislation. In 1990, the Board of Supervisors in San Francisco—the gateway to Silicon Valley, the heart of the world's computer industry—overwhelmingly approved similar workplace regulations, giving local companies with fifteen or more computer operators two years to comply. Again business interests raised an outcry, claiming the regulations would cost over $100 million. They threatened to leave a city already suffering from a severe business downturn, so the mayor and legislators gave in and took significant features out of the regulations, as well as extending the compliance period to four years.

Overseas, particularly in Scandinavia and parts of Europe, the business community, the unions, and the politicians are working together more to assess the extent of the risk and come up with practical, realistic answers with which everyone can live. The pattern is markedly different in America, but the U.S. situation must change. An important factor yet to be felt fully is that this is the first industrial injury in which reporters and editors are at particularly high risk, now that electronic editing systems are universally used in all media categories. There is also a growing tide of behind-the-scenes lobbying building up in influential places, such as the Environmental Protection Agency, where some of the staff feel the need to remedy electromagnetic radiation and chemical pollutants in homes, offices, and other workplaces.

Medical concern is mounting also as the limited research that has been conducted moves from obscure scientific journals onto center stage in more influential publications and is picked up by the general media.

Fuel will be added to the fire by commercial interests, now positioning themselves to exploit the issue. Billions of dollars in potential incremental revenue stand to be generated from the computer hardware market if the replacement cycles for video monitors can be accelerated by concerns about radiation emissions and eyestrain. Several companies are developing low-emission-level monitors—including the industry giants IBM and Apple Computer. In Sweden, monitors incorporating health protection features have been compulsory for some time.

Of course no manufacturers, however actively developing "safer" hardware, will admit any likelihood that their existing products are harmful. The potential for liability claims is enormous. However, there will be no such inhibitions on companies going into the monitor business for the first time, starting up with low-emission-level designs.

Companies pushing forward with liquid crystal display technology have much to gain from this move toward low-radiation hardware.

During the 1980s, this sector had its market horizons limited largely to portable computers and special video display needs where the higher cost of LCDs over CRTs could be justified. Now there is the possibility that, over the next decade, every existing CRT monitor will be a candidate for replacement by an LCD panel or other "safer" alternative. A very powerful lobby is emerging with enormous opportunities to profit from tough computer workplace regulations.

So it is inevitable that there will be a mounting tide of publicity to motivate employees to expect their employers to act positively to protect them from the potential dangers of prolonged periods of computer work. The business community may temporarily stave off both local and federal regulations requiring adjustable workstations, work breaks every two hours, and health training programs. But the interim savings in implementation costs and inconvenience required to conform to mandatory requirements could prove false economies when weighed against the much more severe penalties of increased medical expenses, lost productivity, and employee dissatisfaction.

## Regulations and Standards Needed

We cannot afford to wait for conclusive evidence either way about electromagnetic radiation from video display terminals. We have more than enough evidence already that prolonged repetitive work creates stress and microtrauma, which probably pose a far greater health hazard. Now is the time to adopt regulations to protect employees.

Repetitive stress already ranks as our number one cause of industrial injuries, and there are few people more prone to it than computer operators sitting for long periods without breaks, with bad posture, hitting keys thousands of times every hour.

Yet still we see employee publications—including corporate employee manuals, which can come back to haunt you in court—maintaining that there are no dangers. The future legal liability consequences for any business not showing *now* at least some concern for its computer operators could be enormous.

But the threat of litigation should not be our prime motivation for planning against the contingency that computers may be confirmed as the specific cause of a number of health problems. The basic precautions to protect both computer operators and the corporate cash reserves need not be either complex or costly for management to intro-duce without delay. Their cost may even benefit the bottom line by increasing productivity and reducing the expenses of sick leave, medi-cal treatment, and staff turnover.

A sensible first step is to formulate—and promulgate—a corporate policy statement. It should put much of the responsibility for healthy computing where it belongs—with the people who actually use the computers. The policy could run along the following lines:

### Draft Policy Statement

The company shares the concerns that many of our employ-ees feel as a result of recent publicity about potential health problems from prolonged and extensive operation of com-puters.

Much of the limited authoritative medical and scientific opinion available at this time is inconclusive and contradicto-ry. Particularly uncertain is the potential for harm from electrical and magnetic forces generated by power lines, electric blankets, television sets, clocks, and other electrical devices, as well as by computer monitors.

The consensus of expert opinion is that working at comput-ers need not pose any exceptional medical hazards and need not be in any way detrimental to health *if the operators themselves ensure that they work comfortably and sensibly.* The following guidelines are designed to ensure your safety when using a computer.

- Adjust your chair and working position so that your feet can rest on the floor and, when sitting upright, your fingers fall naturally to the keyboard with your arms and hands in a sightly downward slope. There should be no sharp angles at your wrists.
- Adjust the monitor so that it can be viewed comforta-bly at, or slightly below, eye level. Use a shade or adjust the monitor or the lighting to avoid distracting reflections in the screen. Sit at least two feet away from the front of the monitor, and avoid working for prolonged

periods within about three feet of the back or sides of a monitor.
- Change your position frequently, taking opportunities to stretch and move your arms, head, neck, shoulders, legs, and back. Stand up and move around for a brief period every ninety minutes. Use any breaks from the keyboard to stand and stretch.
- Blink regularly and use mild artificial solutions if your eyes feel dry and uncomfortable. This condition is usually caused by blinking at a lower than normal rate when concentrating on the screen, so the eyes temporarily lack natural lubrication.
- Keep the computer screen, and your glasses if you wear any, clean from both dust and smears. If you feel you are suffering from eyestrain, have your eyes examined professionally. You may need a new prescription, or have a vision problem not associated with your work.
- It is particularly important for those doing any kind of sedentary work, such as data processing, to exercise, follow a sensible diet, and drink plenty of water. Probably the most useful things you can do to protect your health is to avoid excess consumption of junk food, severely restrict your intake of sugar and stimulants, such as caffeine, and drink at least six glasses of water and walk for about half an hour every day.

If you have any questions, or need help in making your work environment more comfortable, please consult your supervisor.

## Audit Your Risk

The issuing of such a policy statement should be accompanied by an audit or survey of the situation within the organization. This should lead to a detailed briefing on the subject for supervisors and line management. They should then be sufficiently well informed to identify particular problems within their areas of responsibility and be able to answer questions from subordinates. Discuss the policy also with union and employee representatives through your established consultative procedures.

An audit of your corporate vulnerability to computing-related health problems can pay big dividends. It will help to identify your potential exposure to liability claims, employee dissatisfaction, and negative publicity. You may well find that the cost of instituting such changes as adjustable workstations, periodic rest breaks, and a modest training program is highly cost-effective in improving productivity and morale.

The need for such expensive measures as replacing conventional CRT monitors with special low-electromagnetic-emission types is far from proven at this time. But the benefits to computer operators of being able to adjust and control their own working positions, particularly relative to the screen and keyboard, can no longer be disputed. It is particularly important when the same computer workstation is used by different employees who range considerably in size and work position preferences. It should be cost-effective to build a high degree of adjustment into any workstation that is used by two or more different shifts during a twenty-four-hour period.

Employees have good grounds for complaint if monitors cannot be adjusted easily to at least a limited extent. Most now come with swivel and tilt stands built in, and such stands are also available as accessories from about $20. A better range of movement is provided by articulated arms that fasten to the desk or wall and support the monitor above desk level. Prices in quantity or from discount suppliers start at about $50.

Many of the protective screens marketed to put in front of video displays are of questionable value for protection from electromagnetic radiation, but most do a reasonable job of reducing glare and unwanted reflections. Their provision demonstrates the employer's concern for the welfare of operators, but they should not be considered a substitute for advising operators to sit at least two feet back from the monitor.

The NoRad Shield shown in Figure 11 is an example of a good-quality screen shield that can protect against certain forms of electrical radiation from the front of computer monitors, as well as reduce glare and unwanted light reflections.

One of the best precautions an employer can take is to keep well informed of the mounting public and computer industry debate on this whole issue of potential health hazards. It makes sense to add the topic

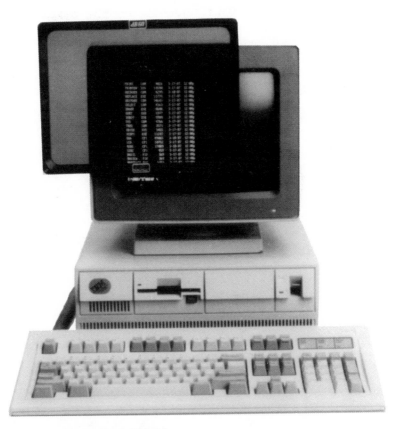

**Figure 11.** The NoRad Shield.

to management clippings and other ongoing news monitoring services. One effective way of keeping in touch is to do a monthly updating search for computer health reports on databases such as the Dow Jones News or *Financial Times* news services.

International organizations need to keep in touch with what is happening in other countries, and the European media are particularly important sources for computer health coverage.

Corporate contingency planning should also include assigning specific managers in the legal, medical, and data processing specialities to keep watching briefs and alert senior managers, particularly in legal and human resources, of important developments.

This may seem outside the normal sphere of contingency planning for emergency situations, but a sudden epidemic of liability claims by data processing operators, or actual work stoppages, could be as disruptive and damaging as fire, flood, or earthquake.

# 11

# VDT Radiation: Is It Really Dangerous?

There is one potential danger to your health from using a computer that might be fatal. But we probably will not know until the late 1990s whether the electrical and magnetic radiation from our video monitors causes cancer, cataracts, or birth defects or affects our health in other ways. In this vacuum of scientific knowledge, we have the hard-earned lessons of asbestos and tobacco to warn us to take some basic precautions.

We *do know* already that our monitors are not bombarding us with microwaves or with sufficient intensities of X rays or other powerful ionizing radiation to cause obvious short-term damage to living cells. That suggests there is no cause for immediate panic.

But we *do not know* if our protracted exposure to the low levels of electrical and magnetic radiation from our monitors has a cumulative damaging effect similar to microtrauma and repetitive stress injury. This radiation may prove to be insignificant and harmless. Unfortunately, there are enough indications of *possible* dangers to merit all computer users' taking the VDT radiation issue seriously. We cannot rely on past assumptions or on glib reassurances from those with commercial interests to protect.

## Strong and Weak Fields May Be Harmful

It was long assumed by scientists that strong electrical and magnetic fields do not have detrimental biological effects on our bodies. Now there is growing belief in links between cancers and other health problems among children, pregnant women, and workers who have been exposed to the strong fields emanating from electrical power lines and transformers.

Scientists are also taking a fresh look at long-held assumptions about the safety aspects of small and weak electrical and magnetic fields. Research now indicates the possibility that small electrical and magnetic pulses of energy radiated by cathode ray tube VDTs may have biological effects. They may, for example, affect the molecules of enzymes in our bodies that play an important role in metabolic processes.

Research at the Massachusetts Institute of Technology and the National Institute of Standards and Technology points to the possibility that faint electric fields could result in a cumulative buildup of certain chemicals in our cells.

Any environmental factor that might cause unnatural changes in cell structure or activity *must* be taken seriously. Consequently it makes sense, especially as computer users, to limit our exposure to radiation from any electrical equipment.

## Electronic Smog

All electrically powered devices emit radiation of different types, at widely differing degrees. So in developed countries we live in the middle of a kind of electromagnetic smog. Our environments are polluted with radiation from power lines, transformers, and other electrical equipment. The VDT is only one of over 10,000 possible sources of electromagnetic radiation that we may encounter in our normal work and leisure activities.

However, the computer monitor is a source of both electrical and magnetic radiation, to which many of us are increasingly being exposed at close proximity and for excessively long periods. If this radiation has the capacity to hurt us, we are presenting ample opportunities for it to do so.

We have to keep this issue in perspective. Your VDT probably presents no significant risk if you sit a couple of feet away from it and do not use it on average for more than four hours a day. Even the heaviest computer use is probably not as damaging as sleeping regularly under an electric blanket. But nobody knows for sure, and a great deal of misinformation is being distributed. There are very powerful commercial forces at work. Employers and the manufacturers of VDTs could face enormous liability consequences if it is proven that the some 100 million VDTs currently in use cause cancer or cataracts. On the other side of the coin, fortunes are to be made from marketing devices that ease computer-user fears about the possible hazards posed by their VDTs.

Whatever the facts, we cannot ignore the possibility that the low-frequency electromagnetic radiation and other force fields set up by components in our computers and VDTs may be very hazardous to both our physical and mental well-being. By using the information that follows and by keeping abreast of developments as they are reported in the media, you can analyze your degree of potential risk and take the simple measures available to protect yourself. In particular, this issue should not be ignored when computers are used intensively by young people, the elderly, or women of childbearing age. Also pay special attention if you have older monitors—particularly color displays—which may be malfunctioning and emitting greater than normal radiation.

But above all, don't panic. There appears no need to rush out and buy an expensive "low radiation" monitor or one of the enormous variety of "protective shields" now hitting the market as entrepreneurs exploit public concerns about VDT radiation hazards.

## Lead Aprons and Other Barriers

Some computer users have even been frightened into wearing lead aprons of the type used during X-ray examinations. Let's tackle that nonsense immediately. The potential problem is not from X rays at all, but from electromagnetic radiation, against which lead shields, or even concrete walls, are not effective. Indeed, as lead aprons are heavy and tend to be uncomfortably hot, wearing one for long periods while computing could in itself be very detrimental to your health!

In fact, there is no practical barrier that you can put up between yourself and your VDT that will protect you from all the electrical and magnetic fields that are the cause of concern. However, the strength of these fields does fall off significantly over even short distances. So sitting well back from the screen dramatically reduces your exposure to radiation—and is good for your eyes and your posture also.

---

## Quick Fix #26

Adjust the layout of your workstation so that you are forced to sit well back from the monitor. You should not be able to touch the screen when you are sitting correctly at the keyboard.

Congratulations! You have now reduced your exposure to electrical and magnetic radiation to levels that are probably safe. (You may also find that you have eased lots of physical stress and strain because your posture has improved now that you are not sitting hunched up to the screen.)

---

## Does Adjusting the Screen Display Reduce Radiation?

No. Turning down the brightness or contrast controls will not reduce the amount of radiation emitted. You may slightly prolong the life of your monitor by having a dim picture, but this can be as detrimental to your eyes as having a screen image that is excessively bright.

You will not derive any meaningful health benefits either from the popular software utilities that blank or dim your screen after a few minutes if the computer is not being used. They may help to prolong the life of the monitor, but dimming the screen does not significantly reduce the radiation it emits.

The healthiest habit, if you are not going to use the computer for some time, is to move farther away from the monitor or switch it off. Some people put their monitors on swiveling articulated arms that enable the VDT to be pushed well away when not needed.

Another way to reduce radiation exposure is by having two distinct and separate work surfaces—one for computing tasks and the other for working with papers or at other noncomputing tasks.

## But Will I Damage My Monitor If I Switch It Off?

If you are an older motorist, you will remember the old advice to warm up your car engine before driving off. Now we are told that automotive technology demands that we not idle our engines, but get moving straight away.

The technology for electrically powered equipment has changed also, and we now have to adjust to the concept of machines that do not "wear out" in the conventional sense from continual use. Moreover, preserving human health is far more important than achieving probably minor and even debatable improvements in the operating life of computer monitors.

The standard technical advice to computer users is to not switch

℞

# Quick Fix #27

Check to see if you or your family or colleagues are being exposed unnecessarily to radiation from computer monitors and other electrical equipment. Is such equipment positioned incorrectly, and left on unnecessarily? (Remember that emissions from the back or sides of a monitor tend to be stronger than those from the front.)

For example, many home computer workstations are backed up against a wall to save space. The radiation from the rear of the monitor might pass through the wall and reach a baby's crib on the other side. In the office, staggering adjoining desks can result in configurations that make workers not using computers more vulnerable to the radiation from the side and rear of a monitor than the person actually operating the computer.

off the monitor, except for long periods of several hours when it will not be needed. Many monitors are never switched off at all—their screens may be dimmed, but they continue perpetually buzzing quietly away—and emitting radiation.

This may slightly increase monitor operational life because the greatest time of stress for almost any electronic device is in the moments when current surges through it as it is switched on. But heat can also stress electronic equipment, so what you gain in one respect may be lost in another. Anyway, from the operator's viewpoint, switching off the monitor (and other electrical equipment that emits radiation, notably laser printers) is the first priority to reduce possibly harmful electrical and magnetic emissions.

## What Causes the Radiation?

Computer monitors are very similar to television sets. The screen you see is one end of a glass tube. At the other end is an electron gun. The beam of electrons generated in this gun are targeted and accelerated toward your end of the tube by a device called a flyback transformer. To enable it to create and vary the display image, the beam is deflected up or down and from side to side by variable magnets called deflection coils.

When the beam hits the phosphor coating on the inside of your end of the glass tube, it causes the coating to glow with the light that you see as a screen display. The display changes as the flyback transformer and deflection coils move the beam in response to instructions from the computer. You hit the key for the number 7, so a 7 appears on your screen as the beam travels across it to refresh the image on the phosphorescent coating.

Although the results of the electronic activity going on inside your monitor appear on the screen at the front, the electronic "muscles" doing the work—the transformers and coils—are mainly at the rear. Consequently, most of the radiation is emitted from the back and sides. You may be well out of any harm's way in front if you are two feet from the screen, but you may need to be four feet away from the back or sides of the monitor.

## Do Screen Shields Stop the Radiation?

Only partially. The main benefit from many shields is not reduced radiation, but a cleaner monitor screen and reduced light glare and reflection.

The radiations from the VDT that concern us are both electrical and magnetic, each being emitted at very low frequencies (VLF) and extremely low frequencies (ELF). Some antiradiation shields are effective at stopping the electrical radiation coming out toward the operator via the end of the glass tube. But you have to ground them properly so that the electrical energy is safely dissipated.

Obviously these shields do nothing about electrical radiation from the back and sides. They also do not block magnetic radiation, which some research indicates may be the cause for most concern. There may also be health problems because of the unique way in which computer monitors expose us to a combination of electrical and magnetic radiation. But that, like virtually everything else in this topic, is not proved.

Most shields are not effective at all against ELF electrical radiation, which some researchers suspect may be the most serious form of radiation from monitors. Unfortunately, there are also many shields on the market that have no merit at all. If they offer any benefits, it may be to reduce unwanted light reflections and glare from the screen. But some can even be counterproductive in that respect, deteriorating the image or causing distracting patterns that raise your stress level and worsen eyestrain.

So buy antiglare and antiradiation shields with great caution and do not assume that any are a substitute for correct lighting or for sitting so that you are at least a full arm's length away from the monitor—the farther the better.

## What About Low-Radiation Monitors?

Be careful also in buying, or persuading your employer to supply, the special monitors that still use cathode ray tubes with their transformers and coils but claim to have significantly lower radiation levels. Some give, as do the antiradiation shields, a distorted perception of safety. At present, monitors that conform to the world's most stringent standards—those developed in Sweden—still cannot be regarded as without risk. But they should at least reduce some of the radiation at the back and sides, as well as in front, so are inherently better than add-on shields.

It promises to be a long time before we have any proper controls or agreed standards for acceptable radiation levels from monitors sold in the United States and most other countries. Our legislators have a strange sense of priorities. Monitors and other electrical equipment are regulated mostly for how their radiation may interfere with other *machines*, notably radio and television receivers. We don't officially care much how the radiation affects people!

The Swedish standards were originally only for VLF emissions, with the ELF requirements due to follow later. They are only guidelines and still need their validity proven conclusively, and they do not cover the possibly more worrisome magnetic radiation. However, they do demonstrate a political concern for computer users that is noticeably lacking in the rest of the world.

If you want a guaranteed safer monitor, you have to move away from conventional cathode ray tube technology to hardware that does not incorporate the coils, transformers, and other electronic devices that generate significant levels of VLF, ELF, and magnetic radiation. That means liquid crystal, electroluminescent, and gas plasma displays. Their development to the point where they will have the versatility and picture quality of conventional CRTs is being accelerated by the concern about radiation emissions. But they are still more expensive and have other drawbacks.

To be realistic about this controversial affair, most of us will continue for years to use monitors that may be seriously hazardous to our health. The most practical advice at this time is at least to keep them at arm's length!

# Index

addiction, 6
airflow, 21–23
airline workers, 4
akido, 12
allergies, 24–25
alpha state, 110
American Ergonomics Corporation,
    114, 121
Apple Computers, 128
Australia, 50–52

backache, 1, 19, 113, 114–115
bilateral carpal tunnel syndrome, *see*
    repetitive stress injury
birth defects, *see* pregnancy
body audit, 16
brain, 14
breathing, 6–7, 13, 79–80, 96

carpal tunnel release surgery, 49, 53
carpal tunnel syndrome, *see* repetitive
    stress injury
chairs, 8–10, 112–123
children, 5–6
circulation, blood, 7, 13, 16, 94–96

color, 26, 99–100
Compushade, 27
Congressional Office of Technology
    Assessment, 101–102
corporate policy statements, 130–131
cosmetics, 23, 244
cost implications, 113–114, 128
Covox, 60

dermatitis, 23
desks, 8–10, 109–110, 112, 123–126
diet, 78–93
    carbohydrates, 85
    cholesterol, 84–85
    eyes, 36
    fluids, 94–96
    food additives, 86–87
    headaches, 47
    menus, 89–93
    protein, 85–86
    stimulants, 80–84
    stress, 88
    sugar, 82–84
    water, 87–88
digestion, 96